I0082416

Spleen Clean

Immunity Boost through Deep Spleen Detoxification

Spleen Clean
Immunity Boost through Deep Spleen Detoxification

Copyright © *Levitas One*, 2024
All Rights Reserved

This book is subject to the condition that no part of this book is to be reproduced, transmitted in any form or means; electronic or mechanical, stored in a retrieval system, photocopied, recorded, scanned, or otherwise. Any of these actions require the proper written permission of the author.

What are the NoMAD Plans?

Developed by Dr Ash Kapoor, the NoMAD Plans represent a transformative approach to health and wellness that combines the wisdom of ancestral practices with contemporary medical insights. The name "NoMAD" not only suggests a journey through the intricate realm of health but also stands for its foundational principles: Nutritional Optimisation, Mindful Adaptation, and Detoxification.

At the heart of NoMAD is the 6 R Framework—Restore, Release, Repair, Renew, Reframe, and Represent. This methodology addresses the root causes of illness, combats chronic inflammation, and cultivates authentic vitality, guiding individuals through a transformative process.

Tailored specifically to each individual, NoMAD journeys are meticulously crafted to rebalance the body, strengthen the mind, and rejuvenate overall health. By integrating ancestral practices with cutting-edge, innovative treatments—all under strict medical oversight—NoMAD Plans offer a personalised pathway to sustainable, long-lasting well-being that resonates with your unique life circumstances.

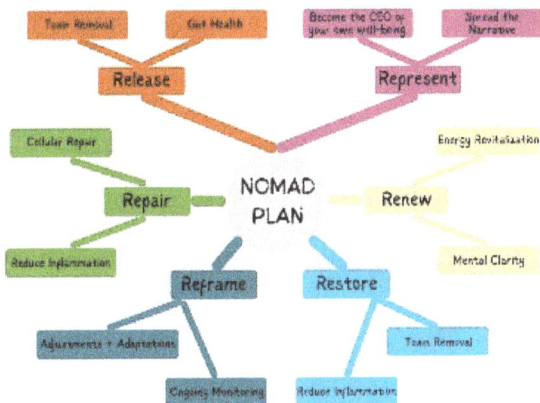

Levitas One:
"As Is In, As Is Out"

Reflecting the belief that our internal well-being is mirrored in our external environment. Founded by Dr Ash Kapoor, Levitas One serves as the vehicle for delivering NoMAD's treatment plans. It envisions a healthcare future where patients are at the centre of a fully integrated, multidisciplinary approach. Guided by Nomads 6 Rs— Restore, Release, Repair, Renew, Reframe, and Represent— Levitas One empowers self-care through personalised guidance and minimal intervention, promoting long-term health, balance, and sustainability.

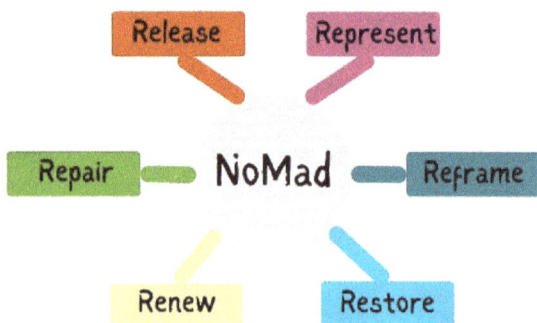

Release Represent

Repair — NoMad — Reframe

Renew Restore

Table of Contents

Preface

My name is **Ash Kapoor** and I have spent nearly 35 years in medical practice, with a growing passion for **regenerative medicine**. This field seeks to harness the body's natural healing processes. Over the course of my career, it has been profoundly enlightening to recognise how, when given the proper nutrition and environment, our organs have an extraordinary ability to serve and protect us. Among these, the spleen plays a particularly vital role, especially in the realm of immune health.

While we have always known the spleen contributes to our immune system, the extent of its influence is often underappreciated. That was certainly true in my experience until I began delving deeper into its functions. Beyond its traditional association with filtering blood, the spleen is intricately involved in **digestion, energy regulation**, and **immune defence**. I came to understand that caring for this organ is crucial for maintaining overall health and well-being.

This book is my attempt to bridge the gap between **ancient wisdom** and **modern innovations**, offering insights into how we can care for and protect our spleen naturally. Drawing from **Traditional Chinese Medicine (TCM)**, **Ayurveda**, and the latest scientific advancements in nutrition and detoxification, this guide will help you understand how to nourish your spleen and enhance its function for optimal health.

Through thoughtful attention to **diet**, **lifestyle**, and **therapeutic practices**, we can support our spleen to perform at its best. I hope this book inspires a renewed appreciation for this essential organ and provides practical tools to help you care for it as naturally and effectively as possible.

Introduction

Importance of Detoxification in Traditional Medicine

Detoxification has long been a cornerstone of traditional healing systems across the globe, from **Ayurveda** to **Traditional Chinese Medicine (TCM)** to **Native American practices**. These ancient systems emphasise removing toxins from the body to restore balance, improve health, and prevent disease.

In TCM, detoxification is often focused on vital organs such as the **liver**, **kidneys**, and especially the **spleen**. The spleen, which plays a crucial role in **blood purification** and **immune function**, is considered the foundation of digestion and energy (Qi) production. By clearing the body of accumulated toxins, people can restore the spleen's natural abilities to filter impurities and support health.

Imagine your body as a car engine. Over time, without regular oil changes and cleaning, the engine becomes clogged with debris, running less efficiently. Similarly, toxins—from **environmental pollution**, **processed foods**, and **stress**—clog our systems, leading to sluggishness, poor immunity, and inflammation. Detox practices act like an oil change for the body, keeping everything running smoothly.

Clinical Case History

A 42-year-old female patient experienced chronic fatigue and bloating for several years. After embarking on a 21-day spleen-focused detox program incorporating TCM principles—using spleen-strengthening herbs and a clean, whole-food diet—she reported increased energy, clearer skin, and improved digestion. Lab results confirmed reduced markers of inflammation, demonstrating how detoxification can make a profound difference in overall health.

The Spleen's Role in Overall Health

1

The spleen, often referred to as the "silent organ" in Western medicine, is anything but quiet in traditional healing systems. In TCM, the spleen is one of the most important organs for **digestive health, immune regulation**, and **energy balance**. It is responsible for transforming the nutrients from food into Qi, the energy that fuels the body.

In Western medicine, the spleen's role is well-defined in its support of the **immune system** and **blood filtration**. It removes old or damaged **red blood cells** and filters out pathogens like **bacteria** and **viruses**, keeping the immune system vigilant and functional. However, when the spleen becomes overwhelmed by toxins or inefficient digestion, its ability to perform these tasks weakens, leaving the body more susceptible to illness.

Think of the spleen as the body's **air filter**. The air filter in a car prevents debris from entering the engine, the spleen filters harmful substances from our bloodstream, keeping the body clean and operating at full capacity. But without regular cleaning or maintenance, both the filter and the spleen become clogged, leading to sluggishness and reduced efficiency. Detoxing the spleen keeps it functioning optimally, just like changing your car's air filter.

Clinical Case History

A 55-year-old male with a history of frequent colds and digestive issues underwent a 14-day spleen detox protocol, including light fasting and herbal support (Triphala and Guduchi). After the detox, his digestion improved significantly, and his immune system became more resilient—he reported not getting sick for an entire winter season for the first time in years.

Why Focus on the Spleen?

Focusing on the spleen during detoxification makes sense because this organ is central to both **digestion** and **immune health**. When the spleen is overworked by poor dietary habits, **environmental toxins**, and **chronic stress**, it struggles to perform its vital functions. This can lead to problems like **poor digestion**, **chronic fatigue**, and a weakened immune system, making you more vulnerable to infections and chronic illnesses.

From a TCM perspective, the spleen is also connected to the emotions. It is said to be influenced by **worry** and **overthinking**. In our fast-paced, mentally demanding world, it is easy for the spleen to become taxed by emotional stress. Focusing on spleen health through detox can not only improve physical health but also help clear mental fog and reduce anxiety.

Imagine the spleen as your body's **battery charger**. If your spleen is weak or burdened with toxins, it can't recharge the body's energy stores effectively, leaving you feeling run-down and tired all the time. A detox for the spleen is like recharging your battery—allowing you to regain vitality, improve digestion, and enhance mental clarity.

Clinical Case History

A 38-year-old woman with chronic digestive issues and frequent bloating reported constant tiredness despite eating a relatively healthy diet. After following a TCM-guided spleen detox, which included eliminating raw, cold foods and focusing on spleen-supporting warm, cooked meals, her energy levels and digestion improved. Within weeks, she noticed a drastic reduction in her bloating and overall fatigue.

Springtime as the Ideal Detox Period

In TCM, spring is considered the optimal time for detoxification, particularly of the liver and spleen. Spring represents renewal and growth, making it the perfect time to **cleanse** and **reset** the body after the stagnation of winter. During the colder months, we tend to eat heavier, richer foods, and our activity levels may decline. This often leads to a build-up of **toxins** and **stagnation** in the body. Spring detox helps us shed the sluggishness of winter and prepare for the lighter, more active months ahead.

Think of your body like a garden that's been dormant during the winter. Spring is when you clear away dead leaves, pull out weeds, and nourish the soil to allow fresh new growth. Detoxifying the spleen during this time helps "clear the soil" of the body, removing the toxins that have accumulated over the months and replenishing the body with nutrients that promote growth and vitality.

Spring detox is especially beneficial for the spleen because this is when the body's natural energy flow is at its peak, allowing for easier elimination of toxins. By supporting the spleen's function during this time, you can **boost digestion**, **reduce inflammation**, and **improve energy levels**.

Clinical Case History

A 45-year-old male, feeling sluggish and bloated after a winter of indulging in heavier foods, underwent a spring spleen detox that included an anti-inflammatory diet, herbal teas, and light fasting. Within a few weeks, his energy levels were revitalised, digestion improved, and his overall sense of well-being was restored, illustrating the power of a seasonal detox to reset the body.

Conclusion of the Introduction

The **spleen** plays a central role in maintaining health, from supporting **digestion** and **immune function** to balancing **energy levels**. Traditional medicine systems like **TCM** have long understood the value of detoxifying the spleen to restore balance and prevent disease. By focusing on **springtime detox,** you're not only clearing out the toxins that build-up over time but also preparing your body to thrive in the months ahead.

In the following sections, we will dive deeper into understanding how the spleen works, the science behind detoxification, and practical approaches like diet, fasting, IV therapy, and more to help you optimise your spleen and overall health.

Summary: Introduction

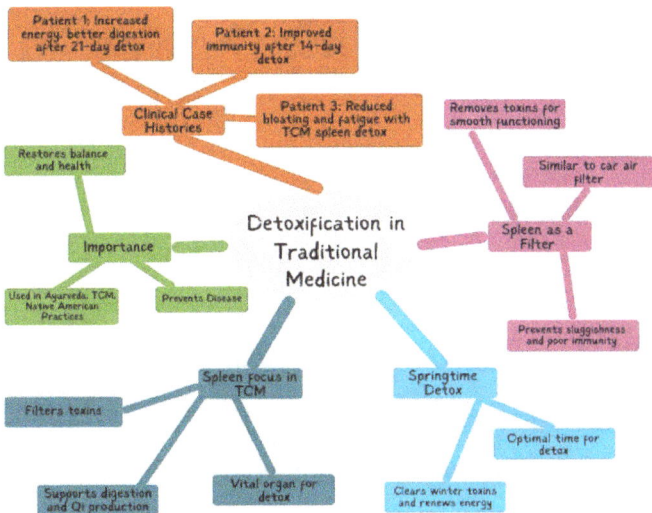

Part 1:
Understanding the Spleen

Chapter 1: Anatomy of the Spleen

Location and Structure

The spleen is a small, fist-sized organ located in the upper left quadrant of the abdomen, protected by the rib cage. Though relatively small, it is the largest organ of the lymphatic system and is part of the circulatory immune system. Its role in maintaining health is significant. It is nestled between the **stomach** and **diaphragm**, surrounded by a network of **blood vessels** that facilitate its blood-filtering functions. Despite its importance, the spleen is often overshadowed by more prominent organs like the heart and liver.

In Western medicine, the spleen is known for its involvement in **blood filtration**. Specifically, it removes old or damaged red blood cells and plays a crucial role in **iron recycling**. It also helps store **platelets**—the cells responsible for blood clotting—and is a critical part of the **immune system**, acting as a reservoir for white blood cells that help fight infections.

To visualise its function, think of the spleen as a **water filter**. Just as a water filter cleans out impurities to ensure the water is safe to drink, the spleen filters out worn-out blood cells and pathogens, ensuring the bloodstream remains healthy and balanced. Without regular filtration, toxins, old cells, and harmful microorganisms would accumulate, leading to systemic inflammation and disease.

Clinical Case History

A 50-year-old male with recurrent infections was found to have a **splenic dysfunction** that was impairing his body's ability to remove damaged red blood cells and pathogens. After undergoing a tailored spleen detox regimen involving diet and herbal support, his spleen function improved, and he experienced fewer infections. Imaging showed improved spleen size and activity, emphasising the organ's importance in immune function.

Spleen in Western Medicine vs. Traditional Chinese Medicine (TCM)

The way the spleen is understood and treated differs significantly between **Western medicine** and **Traditional Chinese Medicine (TCM)**. While Western medicine focuses on the spleen's **physical functions**, like blood filtration and immune support, TCM views the spleen as the centre of **digestion** and **energy production**.

In TCM, the spleen is responsible for transforming food into **Qi**, the body's vital energy. It works in tandem with the **stomach**, which is considered the "cauldron" where food is broken down, while the spleen is the organ that transforms and transports nutrients throughout the body. A healthy spleen ensures that **nutrients** are properly absorbed and converted into energy, keeping the body strong and vital.

In contrast, Western medicine often overlooks the spleen unless it is affected by conditions like **splenomegaly** (an enlarged spleen) or **hypersplenism** (overactive spleen function). For instance, Western medicine recognises the spleen's role in immune response, particularly in clearing infections like **pneumococcus** or **meningococcus**. However, it rarely focuses on preventive spleen health in the way that TCM does, where practitioners work to keep the spleen in balance to prevent **digestive issues**, **fatigue**, and **immunity deficiencies**.

Analogy: Think of the Western medicine view as that of a **firefighter**—only intervening when there's a problem. TCM, on the other hand, is more like a **gardener**, carefully maintaining the health of the spleen throughout life to prevent issues from arising in the first place.

Clinical Case History

A 45-year-old woman suffered from chronic indigestion and fatigue. From a Western perspective, her blood work and spleen size appeared normal, but in TCM, she was diagnosed with **Spleen Qi Deficiency**. Her treatment included **warming foods**, **herbal tonics** like **ginseng** and **ginger**, and **acupuncture.** Within a few months, her digestion improved, and her energy levels returned to normal, highlighting the differences in treatment approaches between Western and Eastern medicine.

Summary: Anatomy of the Spleen

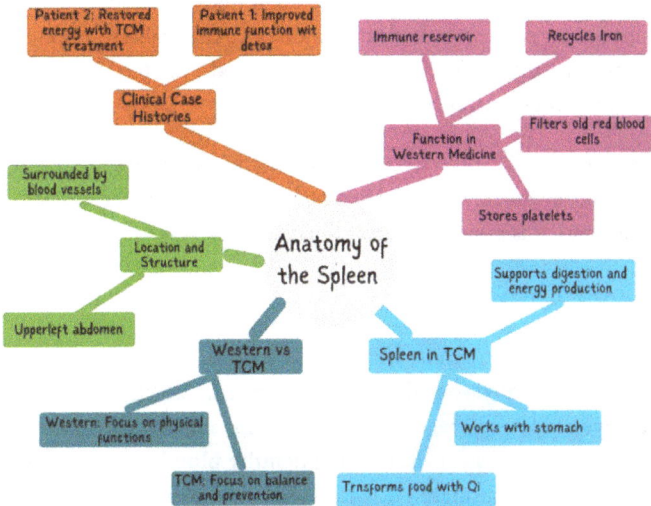

Chapter 2: Functions of the Spleen

Immune System Support

The spleen is a critical component of the **immune system**. It acts as a **blood reservoir**, where it stores **white blood cells** called **lymphocytes** and **macrophages**, which detect and attack pathogens like **bacteria**, **viruses**, and **fungi**. When the immune system detects an invader, the spleen releases these cells into the bloodstream to fight infection.

In many ways, the spleen functions like a **security system**, constantly on alert for harmful intruders. If a harmful pathogen enters the bloodstream, the spleen is one of the first organs to react, activating the body's **immune defences**. Without a well-functioning spleen, the body becomes more vulnerable to infections, especially those involving **encapsulated bacteria**, such as **pneumococcus** and **meningococcus**.

Analogy: Imagine the spleen as your home's security system; if it is broken, intruders can easily enter. Likewise, if the spleen is weakened, it is easier for harmful pathogens to invade the body.

Blood Filtration

One of the spleen's most vital functions is filtering the blood. Every minute, blood flows through the spleen, which meticulously removes old or damaged **red blood cells** and recycles iron. This recycling is crucial for maintaining **healthy blood cell production** and ensuring that there's a balance of oxygen-carrying cells in the bloodstream.

The spleen also acts as a **detoxification organ**, clearing out cellular debris, bacteria, and other harmful substances. In Western medicine, spleen removal (splenectomy) is sometimes necessary due to trauma or disease, but this leaves patients more vulnerable to infections because they lose this essential filtering mechanism.

Clinical Case History

A 60-year-old man with chronic anaemia underwent tests that showed his spleen was holding onto an excessive amount of red blood cells, leading to decreased circulation of healthy cells. After addressing his spleen health through a series of detox protocols, his red blood cell levels stabilised, highlighting the spleen's critical role in blood health.

Energy Metabolism

In TCM, the spleen is viewed as the organ responsible for **energy metabolism**. It transforms the nutrients extracted from food into Qi, the life force that powers all bodily functions. A weakened spleen leads to poor energy production, which manifests as **chronic fatigue**, **poor digestion**, and an inability to fight off infections.

From a Western perspective, energy metabolism is more often linked to **mitochondria** and overall metabolic processes, but TCM uniquely emphasises the spleen's role in converting food into usable energy. When the spleen is overwhelmed with toxins or poor diet, it fails to perform this function effectively, leading to **lethargy** and **digestive sluggishness**.

Analogy: The spleen acts as a quality control department in a factory. It inspects red blood cells and removes any that are defective or damaged, ensuring only high-quality cells are circulating in your body.

Role in Digestion (TCM Perspective)

In TCM, the spleen is at the heart of digestion. It is responsible for extracting the **essence** from food, turning it into energy, and distributing it throughout the body. Poor spleen health leads to symptoms like **bloating**, **gas**, and **poor nutrient absorption**.

TCM practitioners often recommend **warming foods** like cooked vegetables, soups, and broths to support spleen health. Cold, raw foods are believed to harm the spleen by slowing digestion, much like how cold weather can slow down a car's engine.

Clinical Case History

A 35-year-old woman complained of chronic bloating and difficulty digesting raw vegetables. She was diagnosed with **Spleen Qi Deficiency** in TCM and advised to switch to a warm, cooked diet rich in spleen-supporting foods. Within weeks, her digestion improved significantly, showing the connection between diet and spleen health.

Summary: Functions of the Spleen

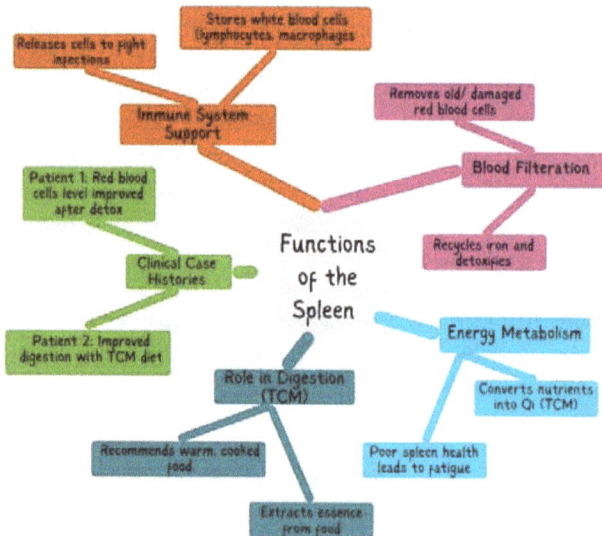

Chapter 3: Signs of an Unhealthy Spleen

Symptoms of Spleen Qi Deficiency

In TCM, **Spleen Qi Deficiency** is a common diagnosis for people experiencing chronic fatigue, bloating, and digestive problems. Symptoms of Spleen Qi Deficiency can also include **mental fog**, **weak muscles**, and a general sense of heaviness in the body.

Inflammation and Its Impact

A poorly functioning spleen leads to systemic **inflammation**, which contributes to various chronic conditions like **autoimmune diseases**, **arthritis**, and **metabolic disorders**. When the spleen can't properly filter the blood, toxins build up, leading to inflammation that affects every organ.

Poor Digestion and Immune Function

Poor digestion is often linked to weakened spleen function. In TCM, the spleen is responsible for converting food into nutrients. When this process is impaired, the body struggles to absorb essential vitamins and minerals, leading to malnutrition and further weakening the immune system.

Conclusion of Part 1

This section explored the anatomy, function, and health significance of the spleen from both Western and TCM perspectives, illustrating how vital this organ is to our overall health. By understanding its roles—whether it is filtering blood, supporting immunity, or managing energy production—we can better appreciate the importance of detoxifying and maintaining a healthy spleen.

Summary: Signs of an Unhealthy Spleen

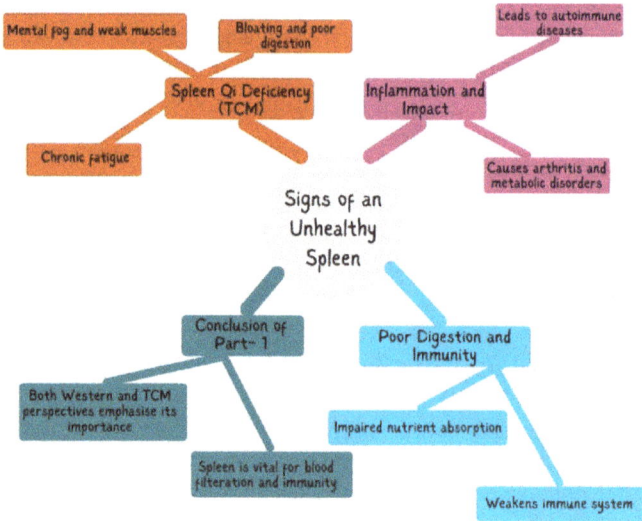

Signs of an Unhealthy Spleen

Spleen Qi Deficiency (TCM)
- Mental fog and weak muscles
- Bloating and poor digestion
- Chronic fatigue

Inflammation and Impact
- Leads to autoimmune diseases
- Causes arthritis and metabolic disorders

Poor Digestion and Immunity
- Impaired nutrient absorption
- Weakens immune system

Conclusion of Part- 1
- Both Western and TCM perspectives emphasise its importance
- Spleen is vital for blood filteration and immunity

Part 2:
Detoxifying the Spleen

Chapter 4: Why Detox the Spleen?

Accumulation of Toxins

Detoxifying the spleen is essential because, over time, the body accumulates toxins from various sources: **pollution, processed foods, chemical exposure**, and even **stress**. The spleen, as a filtration organ, works tirelessly to cleanse the blood of these toxins, but it can become overwhelmed. Just like a vacuum filter that needs regular cleaning, your spleen can become clogged, leading to **sluggishness, inflammation**, and weakened **immune function**.

In modern life, we are constantly exposed to more toxins than our ancestors. The **air we breathe**, the **food we eat**, and even our **personal care products** contain chemicals that can burden the spleen. When the spleen is overworked, it may not efficiently filter the blood, causing **toxins to accumulate** in tissues. This accumulation can lead to symptoms such as **chronic fatigue, digestive problems**, and **weakened immunity**.

Imagine your body as a house and the spleen as the **housekeeper**. If the housekeeper becomes overwhelmed by an excessive amount of dirt and clutter, the house becomes less functional. Similarly, if the spleen is overloaded with toxins, it becomes less efficient at maintaining the health of your blood and immune system. Detoxification helps to **"reset"** the spleen, allowing it to function optimally again.

Clinical Case History

A 40-year-old woman with chronic fatigue and skin rashes underwent a 14-day detox focused on her spleen health. After eliminating processed foods, incorporating spleen-friendly herbs, and using natural detox strategies like fasting, her symptoms improved significantly. Her skin cleared up, and her energy levels rebounded, highlighting the spleen's ability to eliminate toxins when adequately supported.

Link Between the Spleen and Digestion

In Traditional Chinese Medicine (TCM), the spleen plays a critical role in **digestion**. It is responsible for the **transformation** and **transportation** of nutrients, taking what is needed from food and distributing it as energy (Qi) to the rest of the body.

Western medicine often views the spleen as less central to digestion compared to organs like the stomach or intestines, but its role in blood filtration is crucial for maintaining a **healthy digestive system**. When the spleen's filtering capacity is reduced due to an accumulation of toxins, **inflammation** can spread throughout the body, further impairing digestion.

Analogies: Imagine the spleen as a **quality control inspector** in a factory. Its job is to ensure that the nutrients extracted from food are of high quality and that waste is correctly disposed of. If the inspector is distracted or overworked, poor-quality materials slip through the cracks, and waste starts piling up. This is why a sluggish spleen often leads to digestive issues, as it does not correctly regulate nutrient absorption and toxin elimination. The spleen can also be thought of as the **power plant** of the digestive system. It helps convert the raw materials (food) into energy. If the power plant isn't working properly, the whole system runs less efficiently, leading to bloating, fatigue, and poor health.

Connection to Emotional Health

The spleen's health is not only tied to physical processes but also to **emotional well-being**. In TCM, the spleen is linked to the emotion of **worry**. Excessive worry, overthinking, and mental strain can weaken the spleen, leading to digestive disturbances, fatigue, and even **mental fog**. Conversely, when the spleen is healthy and strong, mental clarity and emotional balance are easier to achieve.

Emotional stress can place a significant burden on the spleen. Much like how emotional stress affects the **heart** or **nervous system**, it also disrupts the spleen's ability to transform food into energy. **Chronic stress** and **overthinking** can literally drain the body's energy, leaving the person feeling physically depleted and emotionally overwhelmed.

Analogy: Imagine your spleen as a **battery** that powers both your body and mind. Constant mental strain or emotional stress drains the battery, leaving you with less energy for digestion, immunity, and emotional resilience.

Clinical Case History

A 38-year-old woman with anxiety and poor digestion reported feeling constantly fatigued and bloated. After undergoing a spleen detox focused on reducing emotional stress through **meditation**, **herbal tonics**, and **dietary changes**, she experienced improved digestion, reduced anxiety, and more emotional balance.

Summary: Why Detox the Spleen?

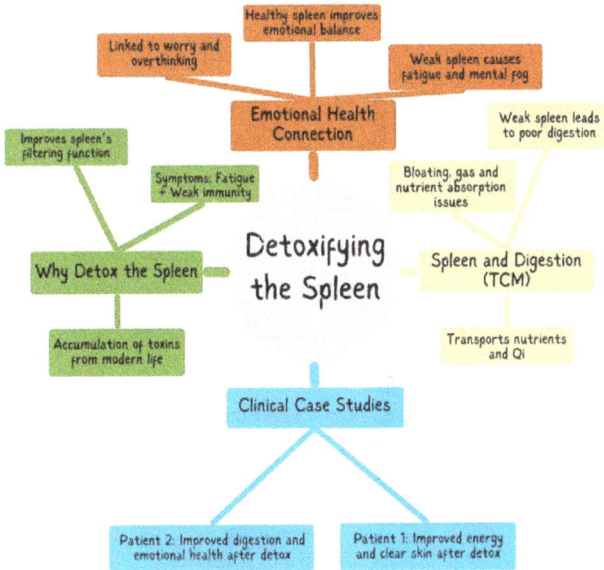

Healthy spleen improves emotional balance

Linked to worry and overthinking

Weak spleen causes fatigue and mental fog

Emotional Health Connection

Weak spleen leads to poor digestion

Improves spleen's filtering function

Symptoms: Fatigue + Weak Immunity

Bloating, gas and nutrient absorption issues

Detoxifying the Spleen

Why Detox the Spleen

Spleen and Digestion (TCM)

Accumulation of toxins from modern life

Transports nutrients and Qi

Clinical Case Studies

Patient 2: Improved digestion and emotional health after detox

Patient 1: Improved energy and clear skin after detox

Chapter 5: The Spring Season and Spleen Health (TCM)

Seasonal Changes and Organ Function

In Traditional Chinese Medicine, each season is associated with specific organs. **Spring** is linked to both the **liver** and **spleen**, making it the ideal time for detoxification of these organs. Spring represents **renewal** and **growth**—a time when the body's energy is naturally more active, facilitating the removal of toxins and revitalisation of organ function.

During the winter months, the body naturally stores more fat and may accumulate toxins from heavier, rich foods. As the energy of spring arrives, the body is primed to shed this burden. Detoxification in the spring aligns with the body's natural rhythms, allowing organs like the spleen to process and eliminate toxins more efficiently.

Think of your body as a **garden**. In the winter, the garden is dormant, but in spring, it is time to **clear away dead leaves** and **prepare the soil** for new growth. Similarly, spring is the best time to clear out toxins and rejuvenate the body for the more active months ahead.

Clinical Case History

A 52-year-old man who suffered from bloating and low energy in the winter months found that a **spring detox** involving warming foods, gentle movement, and herbal tonics restored his energy and improved digestion within weeks, preparing his body for the new season.

Liver-Spleen Interactions

The liver and spleen are closely connected in both Western and Chinese medicine. In TCM, the liver is responsible for the smooth flow of **Qi** (energy) throughout the body, while the spleen is tasked with transforming food into Qi. When the liver becomes overburdened by toxins or stress, it disrupts the spleen's ability to properly metabolise food, leading to **indigestion**, **bloating**, and **fatigue**.

Much like a **team**, the liver and spleen need to work together for optimal health. If the liver is sluggish, the spleen has to work harder to maintain balance, which can lead to further health problems. Detoxifying the spleen without addressing liver health may yield limited results, which is why a holistic approach often involves supporting both organs simultaneously.

Analogy: Imagine the liver and spleen as partners in a **business**. If one partner is overwhelmed and unable to do their part, the other partner has to pick up the slack, which can cause strain on the entire operation.

Clinical Case History

A 47-year-old man with a history of liver inflammation (fatty liver) and digestive issues completed a liver and spleen detox regimen that included **milk thistle**, **dandelion root**, and dietary changes. His liver enzymes normalised, and he experienced improved digestion and increased energy, showing the importance of liver-spleen collaboration in detox.

Best Time for Detox

Spring is traditionally viewed as the **best time for detoxification**, particularly for the spleen and liver. The body's natural rhythms are more aligned with cleansing and renewal during this season, making it easier to release accumulated toxins from the winter months. The increased daylight and warmer temperatures also encourage more **movement**, which supports circulation and detox processes.

In TCM, it is said that the body's energy, or **Qi**, rises with the **spring energy**, facilitating the elimination of waste and toxins. This is why many detox programs are structured around the spring months when the body is most responsive to these processes.

Analogy: Think of your body like a **tree**. In winter, the tree conserves energy, but in spring, it releases its old leaves and grows new ones. The body functions similarly, using spring as an opportunity to release what is no longer needed and begin anew.

Summary: The Spring Season and Spleen Health (TCM)

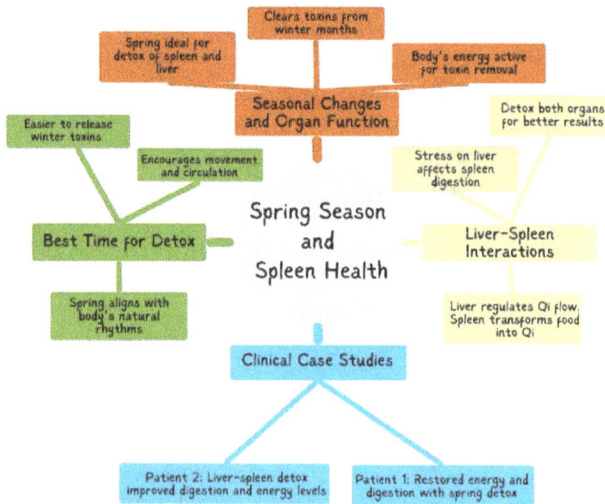

Chapter 6: The Science Behind Detoxification

Modern Research on Detoxification

Modern research supports the idea of detoxification as a means of improving health, particularly in relation to immune function, digestion, and overall vitality. Detoxification involves the process of **removing toxins** that have built up in the body due to poor diet, stress, and environmental exposure. While the liver and kidneys play central roles in detox, the **spleen** assists in filtering blood and maintaining the immune system, ensuring that toxins are removed from circulation.

Studies have shown that regular detoxification—whether through dietary changes, fasting, or herbal supplements—can reduce **oxidative stress**, a major contributor to inflammation and chronic disease. For example, **fasting** has been found to activate **autophagy**, a process in which the body cleans out damaged cells and regenerates new, healthy ones, supporting both the liver and spleen in their detox roles.

Clinical Case History

A 56-year-old woman with chronic inflammation and digestive issues underwent a medically supervised detox program, which included intermittent fasting and antioxidant supplements. After 30 days, her inflammatory markers dropped significantly, and she experienced better digestion, showing the potential of detox to restore balance in the body.

The Spleen's Role in Immune Cleansing

The spleen's function as an **immune organ** makes it critical to the body's detoxification process. By filtering **pathogens** and **damaged cells** from the bloodstream, the spleen helps maintain a healthy balance in the immune system. When toxins build up, the spleen can become overwhelmed, compromising its ability to filter blood efficiently and protect the body from infections.

Detoxification helps the spleen by reducing the **toxic load** it has to process, allowing it to work more efficiently. This also improves overall immune function, making the body more resilient against infections. Regular detox programs support the spleen's blood-filtering role, improving immune response and reducing **inflammatory conditions**.

Analogy: Imagine the spleen as a **traffic cop**, directing the flow of healthy immune cells and removing damaged ones. A detox gives the traffic cop a clearer path, making their job easier and more effective.

Benefits of Seasonal Detox

Seasonal detoxification, especially during the **spring** months, offers numerous benefits, from improved **digestion** and **energy levels** to enhanced **immune function**. When aligned with the body's natural rhythms, detox can help prevent the build-up of toxins, reduce inflammation, and restore overall balance to the body's systems.

In addition to physical benefits, seasonal detox can also improve **mental clarity** and **emotional balance**, as it clears not just physical toxins but also the emotional burdens often associated with the changing seasons.

Clinical Case History

A 42-year-old man reported feeling sluggish and mentally foggy during the winter. After undergoing a spring detox focused on spleen and liver health, including dietary changes and herbal support, he noticed a marked improvement in his energy, mental clarity, and overall well-being.

Conclusion of Part 2

This section explored the reasons for spleen detoxification and its connection to seasonal rhythms, digestion, immune function, and emotional health. By understanding why detoxing the spleen is so important, readers can better appreciate how a well-timed, holistic detox can restore balance, improve digestion, and boost immune health.

Summary: The Science Behind Detoxification

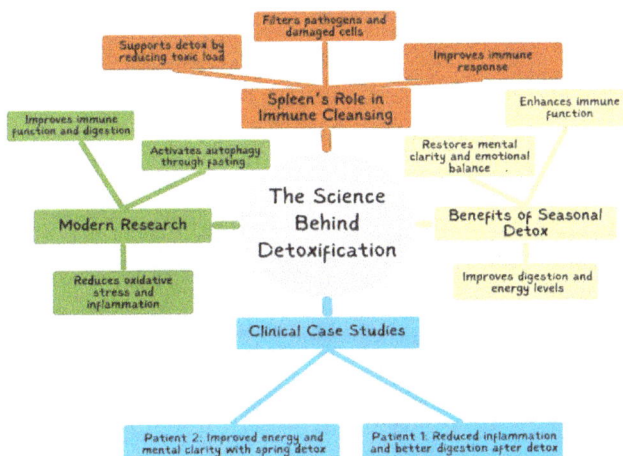

Part 3:
Detox Diet and Nutrition

Chapter 7: Foods That Strengthen the Spleen

TCM Dietary Recommendations

In Traditional Chinese Medicine (TCM), food is considered a primary means to nourish the body and restore balance, especially for organs like the **spleen**, which is central to digestion and energy production. TCM emphasises the importance of **warming**, **cooked foods** to support spleen health, as raw or cold foods are believed to **weaken** the spleen's energy, leading to digestive issues and **Spleen Qi Deficiency**.

One of the core principles in TCM dietary therapy is to focus on **easily digestible foods** that "warm" the digestive system. This includes **soups**, **stews**, **lightly steamed vegetables**, and **whole grains** like **rice** and **millet**. Warm and simple meals are easier on the spleen and promote better **nutrient absorption**. Foods that strengthen the spleen include:

- **Root vegetables** like **sweet potatoes, carrots,** and **parsnips** which provide grounding and nourishing energy.

- **Whole grains** such as **millet, quinoa,** and **brown rice** which offer sustained energy and support the spleen's ability to transform food into Qi.

- **Warming spices** like **ginger, cinnamon**, and **turmeric** can improve circulation, support digestion, and enhance the spleen's energy.

In TCM, it is also recommended to avoid **dairy, excess sugar,** and **cold drinks** as they are thought to create **dampness** in the body, which can overwhelm the spleen and lead to stagnation. Dampness can manifest as bloating, heaviness, and poor digestion.

Clinical Case History

A 40-year-old man with chronic bloating and fatigue switched to a TCM-recommended spleen-nourishing diet. By incorporating warming, cooked foods and avoiding cold, raw meals, his digestive symptoms improved, and he regained his energy, illustrating the power of a proper diet in supporting spleen health.

Seasonal Foods for Spring

Spring is a time of renewal and growth, making it the perfect season for detox and rejuvenation. In both TCM and Western holistic health, eating **seasonal foods** is encouraged to align with the body's natural rhythms. Seasonal, local foods are often rich in the nutrients needed to support **spring detox** and **spleen health**.

For spring, focus on **light, fresh,** and **green** foods to help clear out the heaviness accumulated from winter. Some great spleen-friendly foods for spring include:

- **Leafy greens** like **spinach, kale,** and **chard**. These greens are rich in antioxidants and chlorophyll, which help cleanse the liver and support digestion.

- **Asparagus** and **artichokes** which are gentle on the digestive system and act as natural diuretics, helping the body flush out excess fluids and toxins.

- **Spring onions** and **leeks** are warming and mildly stimulating to the digestive system, helping promote good circulation and digestion.

In TCM, the spring season corresponds to the **wood element**, which is linked to the liver and spleen. Eating foods that support the **liver's detox function** also benefits the spleen, as these organs work in tandem. Foods like **dandelion greens, parsley,** and **beets** help support both liver and spleen health by promoting the elimination of toxins and increasing circulation.

Analogy: Just as you would **spring clean** your home by airing out the space and clearing away clutter, eating light, fresh foods during spring helps cleanse and renew your body, preparing it for the more active months ahead.

Spleen-Friendly Superfoods

Certain superfoods are particularly beneficial for spleen health, as they help the spleen perform its blood-filtering and energy-transforming functions more effectively. These superfoods are nutrient-dense and often rich in antioxidants, supporting overall detox and spleen vitality.

- **Goji berries**: Known for their powerful antioxidant properties, goji berries help protect cells from damage and support healthy immune function. In TCM, they are considered a spleen tonic, helping to nourish Qi and blood.

- **Pumpkin**: A warming vegetable in TCM, pumpkin is easy to digest and supports spleen health by providing vital nutrients without overwhelming the digestive system.

- **Bone broth**: Rich in minerals and collagen, bone broth is considered a spleen-strengthening food. It supports **gut health**, improves nutrient absorption, and helps heal the lining of the digestive system, making it easier for the spleen to do its job.

Incorporating these superfoods into your diet, particularly during detox, can help nourish the spleen and provide the nutrients it needs to thrive. They are especially helpful in reducing **inflammation** and promoting **energy balance**.

Summary: Foods That Strengthen the Spleen

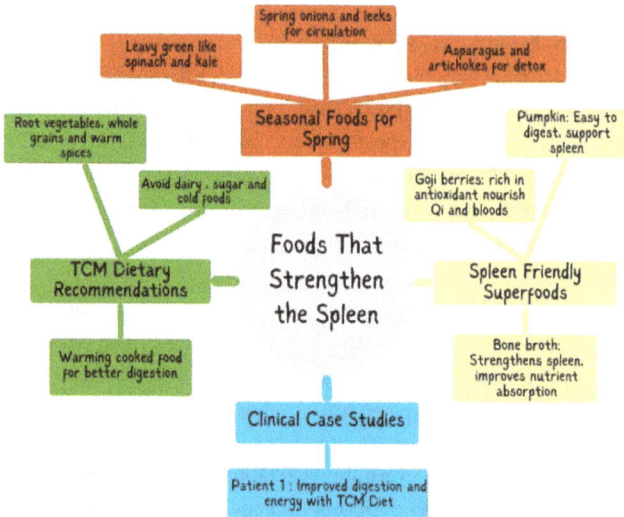

- Spring onions and leeks for circulation
- Leavy green like spinach and kale
- Asparagus and artichokes for detox
- Root vegetables, whole grains and warm spices
- **Seasonal Foods for Spring**
- Pumpkin: Easy to digest, support spleen
- Avoid dairy , sugar and cold foods
- Goji berries: rich in antioxidant nourish Qi and bloods

Foods That Strengthen the Spleen

- **TCM Dietary Recommendations**
- **Spleen Friendly Superfoods**
- Warming cooked food for better digestion
- Bone broth: Strengthens spleen, improves nutrient absorption
- **Clinical Case Studies**
- Patient 1 : Improved digestion and energy with TCM Diet

Chapter 8: The Ultimate Spleen Detox Diet Plan

7-Day Detox Plan

A 7-day detox plan focused on the spleen emphasises **clean eating**, **hydration**, and **gentle fasting** to allow the spleen to rest and rejuvenate. The goal is to reduce the burden on the spleen by providing easily digestible, nutrient-rich foods while eliminating processed foods, sugars, and anything that can create stagnation in the body.

Day 1-3

Start with simple, **liquid meals** like **bone broth, vegetable soups**, and **herbal teas**. These will give your digestive system a break while still providing essential nutrients. Drink **ginger tea** throughout the day to aid digestion and keep the spleen warm.

Day 4-5

Transition to light, solid meals like **steamed vegetables, quinoa**, and **millet**. Avoid raw or cold foods, as they can dampen the spleen's energy. Continue drinking warm teas and plenty of water to flush toxins out of the system.

Day 6-7

Incorporate **probiotic-rich** foods like **sauerkraut, kimchi**, and **miso soup** to promote gut health. This will further support spleen function, as a healthy gut is essential for good digestion and nutrient absorption.

Clinical Case History

A 35-year-old woman with bloating and sluggish digestion followed a 7-day spleen detox plan, focusing on broth and light, warm foods. By the end of the week, her bloating was significantly reduced, and she reported feeling lighter and more energised.

14-Day Extended Detox Guide

For those who want to deepen the detox process, a **14-day extended plan** offers more time to allow the body to fully reset. The first 7 days follow the same plan as the initial detox, but in the second week, you gradually reintroduce more solid foods while continuing to emphasise foods that nourish the spleen and support detox.

Days 8-10

Continue with **cooked grains** like millet and brown rice, along with lightly steamed or sautéed vegetables. Start incorporating **protein** in the form of **wild-caught fish**, **organic chicken**, or **lentils**. Avoid processed meats and dairy, as these can clog the digestive system.

Days 11-14

Focus on **fibre-rich foods** to help cleanse the digestive tract. **Lentil soups**, **sweet potatoes**, and **chia seeds** will support the spleen's detox efforts while also promoting gut health. Avoid refined carbohydrates and sugars, as they can burden the spleen.

Throughout the 14 days, it is essential to stay hydrated with **filtered water**, **herbal teas**, and **infusions** like **dandelion tea**, which support liver and spleen detox.

Clinical Case History

A 50-year-old man with high levels of inflammation and poor digestion completed the 14-day spleen detox program. By the end, his digestion had improved, and his inflammatory markers decreased significantly, highlighting the benefits of an extended detox for systemic inflammation.

Recipes for Spleen Clean

Phase 1 (Days 1-3): Simple Liquid Recipes

- Ginger and Carrot Soup:

Ingredients: Carrots, fresh ginger, vegetable broth, olive oil.

Method: Sauté ginger and carrots in olive oil, add broth, and simmer until soft. Blend until smooth.

Benefits: Warming and easy to digest, this soup supports spleen energy and reduces inflammation.

- **Bone Broth:**

Ingredients: Beef or chicken bones, garlic, onion, 15 – 30 ml apple cider vinegar

Method: Simmer bones with water, garlic, and onion for 12-24 hours. Strain and serve warm.

Benefits: Rich in collagen and minerals, bone broth helps repair the gut lining, easing the spleen's workload.

Phase 2 (Days 4-7): Light Solid Recipes

- **Steamed Vegetables with Quinoa:**

Ingredients: Quinoa, spinach, carrots, olive oil, sea salt.

Method: Steam vegetables and serve over cooked quinoa with olive oil and a pinch of sea salt.

Benefits: Provides easily digestible fibre and nutrients without overwhelming the spleen.

Phase 3 (Days 8-14): Fibre-Rich Recipes

- **Lentil and Sweet Potato Stew:**

Ingredients: Lentils, sweet potatoes, onions, garlic, turmeric.

Method: Sauté onions and garlic, add lentils and cubed sweet potatoes, cover with water, and simmer. Add turmeric.

Benefits: Rich in fibre and nutrients, this dish supports digestion and spleen function while gently detoxifying the body.

Summary: The Ultimate Spleen Detox Diet Plan

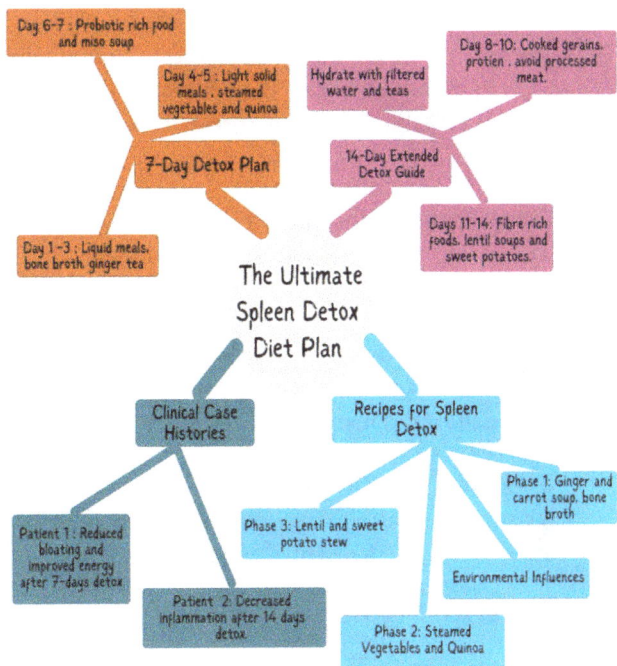

The Ultimate Spleen Detox Diet Plan

7-Day Detox Plan
- Day 6-7 : Probiotic rich food and miso soup
- Day 4-5 : Light solid meals . steamed vegetables and quinoa
- Day 1-3 : Liquid meals. bone broth ginger tea

14-Day Extended Detox Guide
- Day 8-10: Cooked gerains. protien . avoid processed meat.
- Hydrate with filtered water and teas
- Days 11-14: Fibre rich foods. lentil soups and sweet potatoes.

Clinical Case Histories
- Patient 1 : Reduced bloating and improved energy after 7-days detox
- Patient 2: Decreased inflammation after 14 days detox

Recipes for Spleen Detox
- Phase 1: Ginger and carrot soup. bone broth
- Phase 3: Lentil and sweet potato stew
- Environmental Influences
- Phase 2: Steamed Vegetables and Quinoa

Chapter 9: Herbal Remedies for the Spleen

Traditional Chinese Herbs

In TCM, several herbs are known for their ability to **strengthen the spleen** and support detoxification. These herbs are often used in **tonics** or **teas** to help enhance digestion, boost energy, and eliminate dampness.

- **Dang Shen** (Codonopsis): Known as a Qi tonic, it strengthens the spleen and helps improve digestion and energy levels.

- **Huang Qi** (Astragalus): Often used to boost immune function and support spleen Qi, Huang Qi also helps fight fatigue and inflammation.

- **Bai Zhu**: This herb is known for its ability to strengthen the spleen, reduce bloating, and clear dampness, making it ideal for those with digestive issues.

Western Herbal Medicine

In Western herbalism, several herbs support detoxification and spleen function. These herbs are often used in **tinctures** or **supplements** to enhance liver and spleen health.

- **Dandelion Root**: A powerful detox herb, dandelion root supports the liver and spleen by promoting bile production and aiding digestion.

- **Milk Thistle**: Known for its ability to protect and regenerate liver cells, milk thistle indirectly supports the spleen by reducing the toxic load.

- **Nettle**: Rich in minerals and known for its detoxifying properties, nettle supports the body's overall cleansing processes and is a good tonic for the blood and spleen.

How to Use Herbs in Everyday Life

Incorporating these herbs into daily life is simple. You can brew **herbal teas** using **dandelion root**, **ginger**, and **Bai Zhu** to sip throughout the day or take herbal **tinctures** such as **milk thistle** or **Astragalus** before meals. These herbs support digestion, promote detox, and help balance spleen Qi, making them a vital part of any spleen-focused detox program.

Clinical Case History

A 45-year-old woman with digestive issues began incorporating a daily tea made from **ginger, dandelion root,** and **Astragalus**. Within weeks, her bloating and digestive discomfort improved, demonstrating the impact of herbal support.

Conclusion of Part 3

This section has outlined the critical dietary principles and herbal remedies to strengthen and detoxify the spleen. It provides actionable plans and recipes to help readers implement these strategies in their daily lives. By following these recommendations, you can rejuvenate your spleen and improve overall health.

Summary: Herbal Remedies for the Spleen

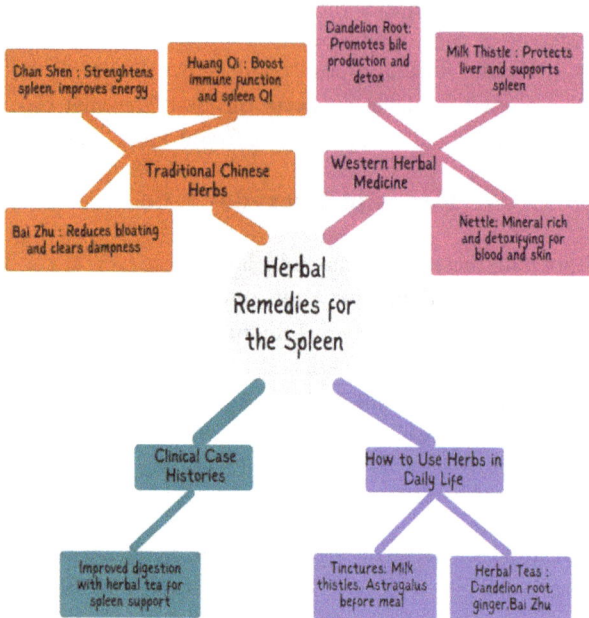

Dan Shen : Strenghtens spleen. improves energy

Huang Qi : Boost immune function and spleen QI

Dandelion Root: Promotes bile production and detox

Milk Thistle : Protects liver and supports spleen

Traditional Chinese Herbs

Western Herbal Medicine

Bai Zhu : Reduces bloating and clears dampness

Nettle: Mineral rich and detoxifying for blood and skin

Herbal Remedies for the Spleen

Clinical Case Histories

How to Use Herbs in Daily Life

Improved digestion with herbal tea for spleen support

Tinctures. Milk thistles. Astragalus before meal

Herbal Teas : Dandelion root. ginger.Bai Zhu

Part 4:
The Role of IV Drips in Spleen Detox

Chapter 10: The Power of Intravenous (IV) Drips for Detox

Overview of IV Therapy in Detoxification

IV therapy, once reserved for hospital settings, is now widely used in holistic and wellness practices to support detoxification and restore nutrient balance. IV therapy delivers nutrients directly into the bloodstream, bypassing the digestive system. This method ensures rapid and efficient absorption of vitamins, minerals, and antioxidants. It is a powerful tool in detox programs, especially for organs like the **spleen**, which plays a crucial role in blood filtration and immune function.

When detoxifying the spleen, IV therapy can be particularly beneficial because the nutrients and antioxidants delivered through IV drips can help reduce **oxidative stress**, eliminate **free radicals**, and enhance the body's ability to process and remove **toxins**. In traditional detox diets or oral supplements, many nutrients are lost in the digestive process. With IV drips, this bypass is a game-changer for those with weakened digestion, poor nutrient absorption, or chronic inflammation.

Imagine the spleen as a garbage disposal that breaks down and eliminates waste products in the blood. Sometimes, the disposal can get jammed or overloaded. IV drips can act like a powerful drain cleaner, flushing out the system and helping the disposal (spleen) work more efficiently.

Clinical Case History

A 60-year-old man with chronic inflammation and fatigue experienced significant improvements in energy and immune function after receiving a series of IV glutathione drips as part of a detox program targeting spleen health. Blood tests showed reduced oxidative stress markers, demonstrating how IV therapy can assist the detoxification process.

How IV Drips Assist the Body's Natural Healing

IV drips provide the body with a **high concentration** of nutrients that are immediately available for use. By delivering essential vitamins, antioxidants, and amino acids directly into the bloodstream, IV drips help boost cellular function, increase energy production, and support the body's natural detoxification pathways. For the spleen, this means more efficient **blood filtration, reduced inflammation**, and better **immune regulation**.

For individuals undergoing detox, IV therapy can be used to provide a quick **nutritional boost** during times when the body's demands for vitamins and minerals may increase. Nutrients like **glutathione, vitamin C**, and **NAD+** enhance the body's ability to eliminate toxins and support liver and spleen health by reducing the oxidative damage that accumulates during periods of heavy detox.

Analogy: Think of IV drips as **power washers** for your body's organs. They provide a direct infusion of essential nutrients to clean out toxins, much like a high-pressure wash clears away stubborn dirt and grime.

The Benefits of Bypassing the Digestive System

One of the greatest benefits of IV therapy is its ability to bypass the digestive system. For those with weakened digestion or compromised nutrient absorption—often the case in individuals with **Spleen Qi Deficiency** or chronic digestive issues—oral

supplements may not be as effective. IV drips deliver nutrients directly into the bloodstream, where they can be used immediately, making them ideal for people undergoing detox or those with weakened digestive health.

During spleen detoxification, IV therapy ensures that the body receives the nutrients it needs without putting additional stress on the digestive system. This is particularly useful when the digestive system needs rest or when nutrients from food may not be properly absorbed due to **inflammation** or poor gut health.

Clinical Case History

A 50-year-old woman with leaky gut and poor nutrient absorption experienced significant improvements in energy and digestion after receiving a series of IV vitamin C and glutathione drips during her detox. The direct infusion bypassed her compromised gut, providing her body with the nutrients needed to accelerate the detoxification process.

Summary: The Power of Intravenous (IV) Drips for Detox

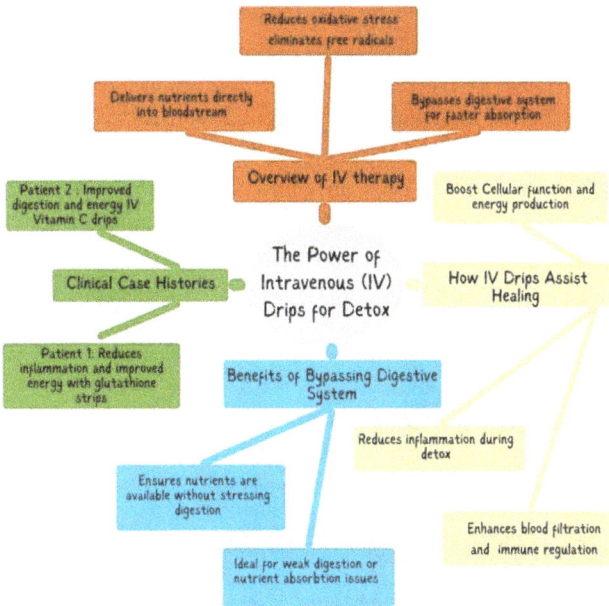

Reduces oxidative stress eliminates free radicals

Delivers nutrients directly into bloodstream

Bypasses digestive system for faster absorption

Overview of IV therapy

Patient 2 : Improved digestion and energy IV Vitamin C drips

Boost Cellular function and energy production

Clinical Case Histories

The Power of Intravenous (IV) Drips for Detox

How IV Drips Assist Healing

Patient 1: Reduces inflammation and improved energy with glutathione strips

Benefits of Bypassing Digestive System

Reduces inflammation during detox

Ensures nutrients are available without stressing digestion

Ideal for weak digestion or nutrient absorbtion issues

Enhances blood filtration and immune regulation

Chapter 11: Key IV Therapies for Spleen Detox

NAD+ (Nicotinamide Adenine Dinucleotide): Cellular Energy and Spleen Health

NAD+ is a coenzyme found in all living cells and plays a critical role in **energy production**, **DNA repair**, and **cellular metabolism**. During detox, NAD+ helps boost the body's ability to repair damaged cells and detoxify the spleen by improving mitochondrial function. When NAD+ levels are increased, the body is better equipped to **eliminate toxins** and regenerate healthy cells.

By supporting **mitochondrial health**, NAD+ improves energy levels, helping to combat the fatigue that often accompanies spleen dysfunction. NAD+ also aids in the repair of DNA damaged by **oxidative stress**, which is critical during detoxification when the body is actively removing harmful free radicals.

Clinical Case History

A 45-year-old man with chronic fatigue and poor digestion completed a 3-week NAD+ IV therapy course as part of his spleen detox plan. He reported improved energy levels, better digestion, and reduced brain fog, highlighting the role of NAD+ in restoring cellular health during detox.

Procaine: Supporting Nervous System and Blood Flow

Procaine is a compound traditionally used as a local anaesthetic, but it has been shown to have regenerative properties, particularly in the nervous system. In IV therapy, procaine helps improve **circulation**, increase **blood flow**, and reduce **inflammation**. This is particularly useful for detoxifying the spleen, as it helps the spleen filter blood more efficiently and improves overall cellular health.

Procaine IV drips can also have a **neuroprotective effect**, supporting the nervous system during detox and reducing the likelihood of inflammation-related discomfort. For those undergoing spleen detox, where energy can be low, procaine helps enhance circulation and nutrient delivery to tissues, promoting faster recovery and more effective detoxification.

Immunity Boosting Drips: Strengthening the Immune Response

IV therapy can be tailored to deliver immune-boosting nutrients such as **vitamin C**, **zinc**, and **selenium**. These nutrients are essential for maintaining a strong immune system, especially during detox, when the body is working hard to eliminate pathogens and toxins. The spleen, as a central organ in the immune system, benefits greatly from an infusion of these nutrients, which can enhance its ability to filter out harmful bacteria and viruses.

Vitamin C, in particular, is a powerful antioxidant that supports spleen health by reducing oxidative stress and improving immune function. High-dose vitamin C IV drips are often used during detox programs to help the body combat inflammation and support immune resilience, particularly during seasonal changes when the body is more susceptible to infections.

Clinical Case History

A 55-year-old woman prone to frequent infections and colds underwent a series of high-dose vitamin C IV drips during her spleen detox program. Following treatment, she reported fewer colds and an overall increase in vitality, demonstrating the importance of immune-boosting nutrients during detox.

Glutathione: The Master Antioxidant for Detox

Glutathione is known as the body's **master antioxidant**, playing a pivotal role in detoxification by neutralising free radicals and supporting liver and spleen function. Glutathione comprised largely of three amino acids: glutamine, glycine, and cysteine, helps remove toxins, including heavy metals, and protects cells from oxidative damage. As part of an IV therapy, glutathione is delivered directly into the bloodstream, providing immediate antioxidant support.

For the spleen, glutathione helps improve its **blood-filtering function** and supports the immune system by protecting white blood cells from oxidative damage. Detox programs often include glutathione IV drips to enhance the body's overall detox capacity, making it easier for the spleen to eliminate waste products and toxins.

Analogy: Think of glutathione as the **detox police force** that goes into the bloodstream, arresting free radicals and removing them from circulation, helping the spleen function more effectively.

PPC (Phosphatidylcholine): Repairing Cell Membranes and Enhancing Detox

Phosphatidylcholine (PPC) is a powerful compound that helps repair cell membranes and improves liver and spleen detoxification. By promoting healthy cell function, PPC supports the spleen's ability to filter toxins from the blood and aids in reducing inflammation. It is especially useful for people with **fatty liver disease** or **metabolic syndrome**, where cellular repair is crucial for recovery.

Clinical Case History

A 48-year-old man with fatty liver and sluggish digestion benefited from PPC drips during his detox program, showing significant improvements in liver function and spleen health.

ALA (Alpha-Lipoic Acid): Powerful Antioxidant Support

Alpha-Lipoic Acid (ALA) is another powerful antioxidant used in IV therapy to support detoxification and reduce inflammation. ALA helps regenerate other antioxidants like **glutathione** and **vitamin C**, amplifying their effects in the body. It also supports the body's ability to process and eliminate toxins, particularly in the liver and spleen.

Analogy: Think of ALA as a **recharge station** for other antioxidants, ensuring that the body's natural detox mechanisms work efficiently and the spleen stays healthy.

Vitamin C IV Therapy: Boosting Immunity and Supporting Detox

Vitamin C, delivered through IV therapy, is a highly effective way to support the spleen during detoxification. High doses of vitamin C can neutralise toxins, reduce inflammation, and support the immune system, which is essential during periods of cleansing. The spleen's immune role benefits from this antioxidant boost, helping the body fight off infections and remove free radicals.

Clinical Case History

A 60-year-old woman undergoing a spleen detox program noticed a reduction in joint inflammation and improved immune function after receiving several high-dose vitamin C IV treatments.

Summary: Key IV Therapies for Spleen Detox

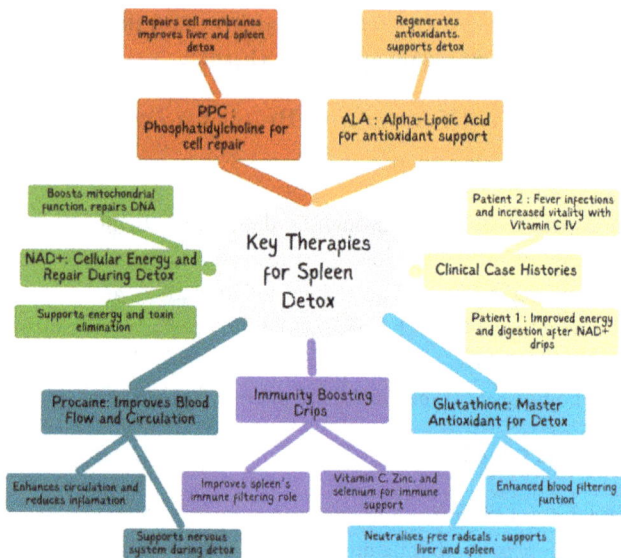

Chapter 12: Integrating IV Drips into a Spleen Detox Protocol

How Often to Use IV Therapy

For most people undergoing a detox program, IV therapy is recommended **1-2 times per week** for optimal results. During an intensive detox, receiving IV drips regularly ensures that the body is consistently replenished with vital nutrients and antioxidants, which helps reduce the toxic load on the spleen. This can vary based on individual needs, detox goals, and overall health status.

For individuals with more significant spleen-related issues, such as chronic fatigue or immune deficiencies, more frequent treatments may be beneficial, particularly in the first few weeks of the detox program.

Combining IV Therapy with Diet and Lifestyle Changes

While IV therapy offers powerful support during detox, it should be used in conjunction with a balanced detox diet and healthy lifestyle practices. A **clean, spleen-friendly diet** that emphasises warming, cooked foods and avoids processed sugars and dairy is crucial for long-term success. Additionally, incorporating **gentle exercises** like **yoga** or **Qi Gong**, along with mindfulness practices like **meditation**, helps keep stress levels in check, further supporting spleen health.

The synergy between diet, lifestyle changes, and IV therapy maximises detox results. While IV drips provide rapid nutrient absorption and detox support, diet and lifestyle help maintain the spleen's health and prevent future toxin build-up.

Safety, Monitoring, and Choosing a Qualified Provider

As with any medical treatment, IV therapy should only be administered by qualified healthcare professionals. It is essential to choose a provider experienced in detox protocols who can tailor IV drips to your specific needs. **Safety monitoring**, including regular blood work, ensures that the treatment is effective and that there are no adverse reactions. Providers will monitor electrolyte levels, hydration status, and overall well-being to ensure that the detox process supports, rather than stresses, the body.

Conclusion of Part 4

This section has explored the various types of IV drips that support spleen detoxification, detailing their benefits and how they fit into a broader detox plan. By using IV drips alongside dietary and lifestyle changes, you can enhance the body's ability to eliminate toxins and support spleen function more effectively.

Summary: Integrating IV Drips into a Spleen Detox Protocol

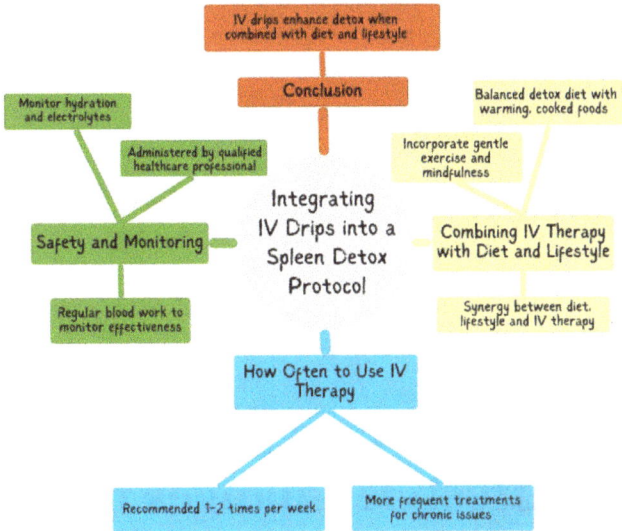

IV drips enhance detox when combined with diet and lifestyle

Conclusion

Monitor hydration and electrolytes

Administered by qualified healthcare professional

Balanced detox diet with warming, cooked foods

Incorporate gentle exercise and mindfulness

Safety and Monitoring

Integrating IV Drips into a Spleen Detox Protocol

Combining IV Therapy with Diet and Lifestyle

Regular blood work to monitor effectiveness

Synergy between diet, lifestyle and IV therapy

How Often to Use IV Therapy

Recommended 1-2 times per week

More frequent treatments for chronic issues

Part 5:
Lifestyle Changes for Spleen Health

Chapter 13: Exercise and Spleen Health

Gentle Exercises for Detox

When detoxing the spleen, it is important to engage in exercises that are **gentle** and **supportive**, rather than those that are too strenuous. During detoxification, the body is working hard to eliminate toxins, so gentle exercises like **walking**, **stretching**, and **light swimming** can encourage circulation without overloading the system.

Gentle exercise stimulates **lymphatic drainage**, which helps the spleen and other detox organs process waste more efficiently. Unlike the cardiovascular system, the **lymphatic system** doesn't have a pump like the heart, so movement is essential for moving lymph fluid throughout the body. By encouraging **gentle movement**, you help the spleen filter toxins from the blood more effectively.

For example, daily 30-minute **walks in nature** are a great way to get the body moving while also reducing stress and boosting circulation. Stretching exercises in the morning and evening can also help improve blood flow, aiding the spleen in its detox process without placing too much strain on the body.

Analogy: Think of gentle exercise as the **broom** that sweeps away debris during a detox. It helps to move waste products out of the body while ensuring that the spleen and other organs aren't overburdened.

Clinical Case History

A 55-year-old man with chronic inflammation and low energy levels incorporated daily walks and gentle stretching during his spleen detox program. After two weeks, his energy increased, and inflammation markers decreased, showing how gentle exercise can complement detoxification.

Qi Gong and Yoga for the Spleen

Qi Gong and **yoga** are ancient practices that align the body, breath, and mind to promote overall health and balance. These practices are particularly beneficial for the spleen during detox. They incorporate **gentle movements** that stimulate the body's natural energy flow (Qi) and support digestion and detoxification.

In TCM, **Qi Gong** is often used to strengthen the **Spleen Qi**, which is essential for digestion and energy production. Certain Qi Gong movements are designed to stimulate the spleen and digestive organs, promoting better circulation and the flow of energy throughout the body. For example, the **"Holding the Balloon"** posture is believed to directly support spleen function by encouraging deep breathing and centring energy in the digestive system.

Similarly, **yoga** postures such as **"Twists"** and **"Forward Folds"** help compress and release the abdominal area, promoting circulation and digestive health. These postures can help move stagnant energy and promote detoxification by gently massaging the organs, including the spleen.

Analogy: Think of Qi Gong and yoga as **internal massages** for the spleen. They gently stimulate circulation and energy flow, helping the spleen do its job more effectively without adding stress to the body.

Benefits of Movement During Detox

Movement during detox has multiple benefits, especially when it comes to supporting spleen health. Exercise, even at a gentle level, helps **increase circulation**, which is essential for the spleen to filter toxins from the blood. When the body moves, it also stimulates the **digestive system**, helping to improve nutrient absorption and waste elimination.

Movement also promotes the production of **endorphins**, which are natural mood enhancers. Since the spleen is connected to emotional health in TCM, supporting a positive mental state through gentle exercise can aid in the detoxification process. Additionally, movement helps reduce **inflammation**, which is often a side effect of toxin build-up in the body.

Regular, gentle movement also helps maintain **muscle tone** and **flexibility**, both of which are important for overall health during a detox. By incorporating low-impact exercises like walking, Qi Gong, or yoga, you ensure that your body is working efficiently to eliminate toxins while maintaining its strength and flexibility.

Clinical Case History

A 42-year-old woman with digestive issues and fatigue found that incorporating daily Qi Gong sessions into her spleen detox plan not only improved her digestion but also increased her energy levels, demonstrating the power of movement during detoxification.

Summary: Exercise and Spleen Health

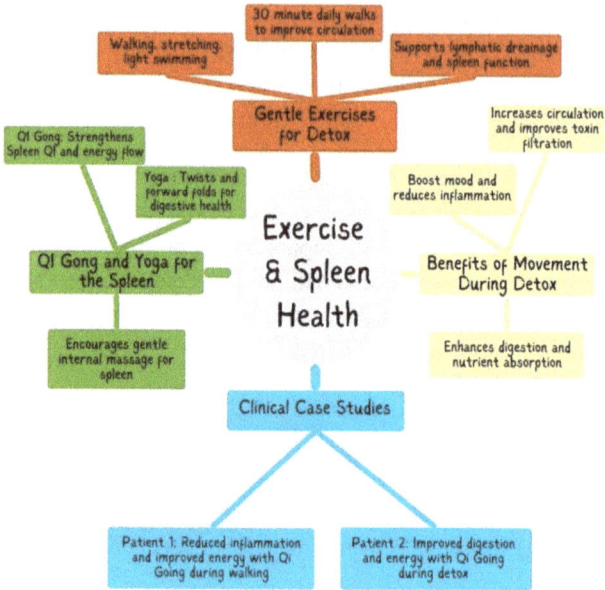

30 minute daily walks
to improve circulation

Walking, stretching,
light swimming

Supports lymphatic dreainage
and spleen function

Gentle Exercises
for Detox

Increases circulation
and improves toxin
filtration

QI Gong: Strengthens
Spleen Qi and energy flow

Yoga : Twists and
forward folds for
digestive health

Boost mood and
reduces inflammation

Exercise
& Spleen
Health

QI Gong and Yoga for
the Spleen

Benefits of Movement
During Detox

Encourages gentle
internal massage for
spleen

Enhances digestion and
nutrient absorption

Clinical Case Studies

Patient 1: Reduced inflammation
and improved energy with Qi
Going during walking

Patient 2: Improved digestion
and energy with Qi Going
during detox

Chapter 14: Managing Stress for Better Spleen Function

The Emotional Connection: Spleen and Worry

In Traditional Chinese Medicine, the spleen is closely linked to the emotion of **worry**. Chronic worry and overthinking can weaken the spleen, leading to **poor digestion**, **fatigue**, and an inability to properly process nutrients. This emotional connection means that managing stress is a critical component of spleen health and overall well-being.

When the spleen is burdened by excessive worry or mental strain, it can lead to **Spleen Qi Deficiency**. This condition manifests in physical symptoms like bloating, fatigue, and food cravings. It is not uncommon for individuals who experience chronic stress or anxiety to also struggle with digestive issues. The spleen, in its role as the body's "**transformer**" of food into energy, becomes less effective when stress disrupts its normal function.

To maintain a healthy spleen, it is vital to reduce sources of worry and practice stress management techniques. A detox program is an ideal time to evaluate emotional stressors and adopt healthier coping mechanisms. By addressing emotional health alongside physical detoxification, you can ensure that your spleen is supported both mentally and physically.

Analogy: Think of worry as a **heavy backpack** that the spleen has to carry around all day. The more you worry, the heavier the load becomes, making it harder for the spleen to function properly.

Stress-Relief Techniques for Detox

Incorporating **stress-relief techniques** into your detox program is essential for maintaining spleen health. Techniques such as **deep breathing exercises**, **progressive muscle relaxation**, and **guided imagery** can help calm the mind, reduce anxiety, and ease the mental burden on the spleen.

Deep breathing exercises are particularly effective because they stimulate the **parasympathetic nervous system**, which promotes relaxation and reduces the body's stress response. By practising 5-10 minutes of deep, diaphragmatic breathing each day, you can help ease the spleen's workload and improve digestion.

Guided imagery involves using mental visualisation to imagine yourself in a peaceful, calming environment. This practice can help reduce mental clutter and relieve stress, allowing your spleen to focus on its detox and digestive roles. Additionally, incorporating **nature walks** into your detox routine is an excellent way to relieve stress, boost circulation, and connect with your body's natural rhythms.

Clinical Case History

A 38-year-old woman with chronic digestive issues and anxiety noticed significant improvements in both her mental and physical health after incorporating daily stress-relief techniques like guided imagery and deep breathing into her detox program.

Mindfulness and Meditation

Mindfulness and **meditation** are powerful tools for supporting spleen health by helping to calm the mind and reduce worry. Both practices involve focusing attention on the present moment, which helps break the cycle of overthinking and anxiety that can weaken the spleen.

Mindfulness practices often involve paying close attention to **breathing**, **bodily sensations**, or **thoughts** without judgment.

This helps to create a sense of calm and balance, reducing the mental strain that can impair spleen function. Even short, 10-15-minute sessions of mindfulness each day can make a significant difference in managing stress during a detox.

Meditation, particularly forms like **guided meditation** or **body scanning**, can help reduce emotional stress and improve the body's ability to detoxify. Studies have shown that meditation can lower **cortisol levels** (the body's stress hormone), which supports the immune system and enhances the body's detox capabilities.

Analogy: Think of mindfulness and meditation as the **reset button** for your spleen. These practices help to clear out mental clutter, allowing the spleen to function more efficiently and effectively.

Summary: Managing Stress for Better Spleen Function

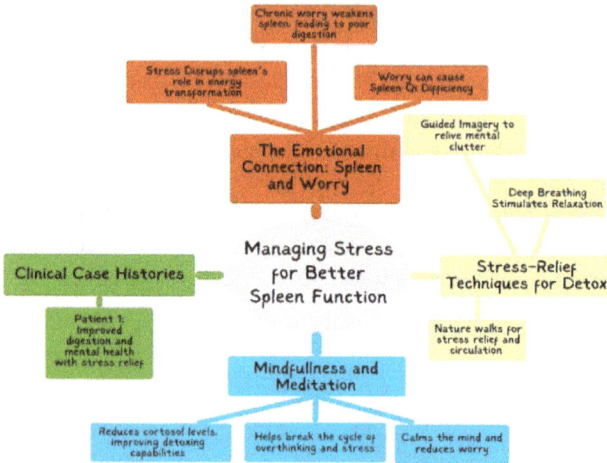

A mind map titled "Managing Stress for Better Spleen Function" with the following branches:

- **The Emotional Connection: Spleen and Worry**
  - Chronic worry weakens spleen, leading to poor digestion
  - Stress Disrupts spleen's role in energy transformation
  - Worry can cause Spleen Qi Deficiency
- **Stress-Relief Techniques for Detox**
  - Guided Imagery to relive mental clutter
  - Deep Breathing Stimulates Relaxation
  - Nature walks for stress relief and circulation
- **Clinical Case Histories**
  - Patient 1: Improved digestion and mental health with stress relief
- **Mindfullness and Meditation**
  - Reduces cortisol levels, improving detoxing capabilities
  - Helps break the cycle of overthinking and stress
  - Calms the mind and reduces worry

Chapter 15: Sleep and the Spleen

The Importance of Rest in Detoxification

Adequate **rest** is one of the most important factors in any detox program, as it allows the body, including the spleen, to heal and regenerate. During sleep, the body performs many of its **detoxification** processes, including repairing tissues, eliminating waste products, and regenerating cells. A lack of quality sleep can impair the body's ability to detox, leaving the spleen overburdened.

The spleen, in particular, benefits from deep, restorative sleep because this is when the body's **immune system** is most active. During sleep, the spleen works to filter the blood, remove toxins, and produce white blood cells that help fight off infection. Without adequate sleep, these processes are compromised, leading to a build-up of toxins and weakened immunity.

In TCM, the spleen is said to function best during the **morning hours**, meaning that getting a whole night of restful sleep allows the spleen to perform its detoxifying duties more effectively during the day.

Clinical Case History

A 45-year-old man with poor sleep and digestive issues noticed significant improvements in both his energy levels and digestion after prioritising sleep as part of his spleen detox plan. His overall sense of well-being improved, underscoring the connection between rest and detoxification.

How Sleep Supports the Spleen's Function

Sleep is the body's natural **recovery time**, during which it undergoes essential processes like **cell repair**, **immune regulation**, and the **elimination of toxins**. The spleen is actively involved in these processes, particularly in its role as a blood filter and immune system supporter. When we sleep, the body shifts from the **fight-or-flight** mode of the day into the **rest-and-digest** state, which allows the spleen to focus on detox and immune function.

During deep sleep, the body produces **cytokines**, which are proteins that help regulate immune responses. The spleen plays a role in storing and releasing these immune proteins, ensuring that the body is prepared to fight infections and heal. A lack of sleep disrupts this cycle, leaving the body vulnerable to toxin accumulation and weakened immunity.

Analogy: Think of sleep as the **night shift** of your body's detox crew. It is when the spleen and other organs get to work, clearing out toxins and resetting the body for the day ahead.

Sleep Routines to Optimise Detox

Establishing a consistent **sleep routine** is crucial for supporting the spleen during detox. Going to bed at the same time each night, creating a relaxing bedtime ritual, and avoiding **stimulants** like caffeine in the evening can help ensure a restful night's sleep.

Incorporating **herbal teas** like **chamomile**, **valerian root**, or **lavender** before bed can also promote relaxation and improve sleep quality. Creating a **calm, dark environment** free from distractions helps signal to your body that it is time to rest, allowing the spleen to perform its essential functions overnight.

Progressive muscle relaxation or **deep breathing exercises** can also be added to your bedtime routine to further reduce stress and prepare the body for rest. These practices help shift the body into a parasympathetic state (rest and digest), where healing and detoxification take place most effectively.

Clinical Case History

A 38-year-old woman struggling with sleep issues and chronic bloating experienced significant improvements in her sleep quality and digestion after incorporating a structured bedtime routine that included herbal teas and relaxation exercises.

Conclusion of Part 5

This section has explored how lifestyle changes, such as incorporating gentle exercise, stress management, mindfulness, and adequate sleep, can support spleen health during detoxification. These practices are essential for reducing mental and physical strain, ensuring that the spleen can perform its detoxifying and immune-regulating functions effectively.

Summary: Sleep and the Spleen

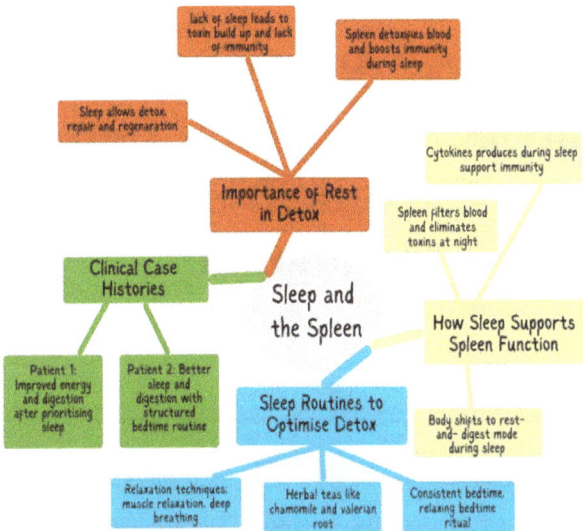

Part 6:
The Role of Spleen Detox in Chronic Disease Management

Chapter 16: Chronic Disease and Spleen Detox

Overview of Chronic Diseases Linked to Spleen Health

Chronic diseases such as **diabetes, autoimmune disorders**, and **metabolic syndrome** have become increasingly common, and many of these conditions are linked to impaired **immune** and **digestive** functions—key roles of the spleen. The spleen's role in **blood filtration, immune regulation**, and **energy transformation** makes it a critical organ for managing chronic diseases. When the spleen becomes overwhelmed by toxins or weakened due to poor diet and stress, the body's ability to fight inflammation, absorb nutrients, and maintain balanced energy levels is compromised.

In Traditional Chinese Medicine (TCM), **Spleen Qi Deficiency** is often associated with long-term digestive weakness, which can exacerbate chronic diseases by leading to **malabsorption, fatigue**, and systemic inflammation. The **immune system** also suffers when the spleen is weakened, as the spleen is crucial for producing and storing **white blood cells** that defend the body against infections and autoimmune reactions.

Clinical Case History

A 50-year-old woman with autoimmune thyroiditis underwent a 30-day spleen detox focused on herbal support, anti-inflammatory foods, and lifestyle modifications. By the end of the detox, her inflammation markers had significantly dropped, and she reported fewer autoimmune flare-ups, highlighting the spleen's importance in managing chronic inflammation.

Detox and Inflammation Control: The Role of the Spleen in Reducing Systemic Inflammation

Chronic inflammation is a hallmark of many diseases, from **arthritis** to **cardiovascular disease**. The spleen plays a critical role in controlling inflammation by filtering blood and removing damaged cells, toxins, and pathogens that trigger inflammatory responses. When the spleen is unable to effectively perform these functions, **systemic inflammation** increases, further damaging tissues and organs.

Detoxing the spleen can reduce **inflammatory markers** in the blood, easing the burden on the immune system. By clearing out accumulated toxins and supporting the spleen's ability to filter blood, detox programs help reduce the inflammatory triggers that drive chronic disease.

Modern research shows that reducing oxidative stress—another contributor to inflammation—can be achieved through detoxification methods such as **fasting**, **antioxidant supplementation**, and **herbal remedies**. These detox strategies can help restore the spleen's filtering capacity, allowing it to better manage inflammation.

Analogy: Think of inflammation as a **fire** in the body. The spleen acts as a **fire extinguisher**, removing the harmful toxins and damaged cells that fuel the flames. A detox helps replenish the spleen's resources, making it more effective in controlling the fire.

Metabolic Syndrome and the Spleen: Detox Strategies for Managing Blood Sugar, Lipid Profiles, and Obesity

Metabolic syndrome, characterised by **high blood sugar**, **elevated cholesterol**, and **obesity**, is another condition in which spleen detox plays a crucial role. The spleen's role in digestion and energy metabolism directly impacts **blood sugar regulation** and **fat**

storage. When the spleen is functioning optimally, the body can efficiently break down food and distribute nutrients, preventing the build-up of excess fats and sugars in the bloodstream.

A spleen-focused detox can help improve **insulin sensitivity**, regulate blood sugar levels, and support weight loss by improving digestion and reducing the body's toxic load. Detox strategies such as a **low-glycaemic diet**, **intermittent fasting**, and herbal support (e.g., **berberine** and **bitter melon**) can help balance blood sugar and reduce the risk of metabolic syndrome.

Clinical Case History

A 48-year-old man with prediabetes and high cholesterol completed a 14-day spleen detox plan, incorporating bitter melon and a low-glycaemic diet. By the end of the detox, his fasting blood sugar levels had decreased, and his cholesterol improved, demonstrating the impact of detox on metabolic health.

Autoimmune Diseases: Supporting the Immune System Through Spleen Detox

Autoimmune diseases, in which the immune system mistakenly attacks healthy tissue, are closely linked to spleen health. The spleen regulates immune responses, and when detoxified, it can help **balance immune activity**. Detox programs that focus on reducing inflammation, supporting immune function, and clearing toxins can help alleviate autoimmune symptoms by giving the spleen the resources it needs to regulate the body's defence mechanisms more effectively.

Clinical Case History

A 35-year-old woman with lupus reported reduced joint pain and fewer autoimmune flares after a 30-day detox program focused on spleen health, showing the connection between detox and immune balance.

Summary: Chronic Disease and Spleen Detox

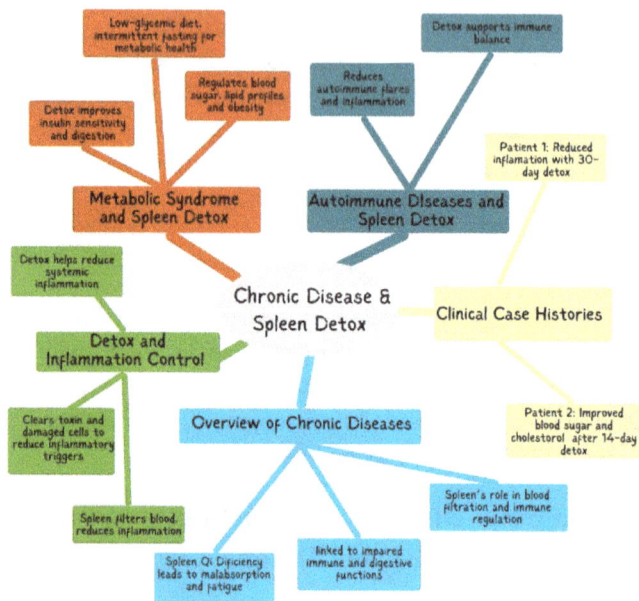

Chronic Disease & Spleen Detox

Metabolic Syndrome and Spleen Detox
- Low-glycemic diet, intermittent fasting for metabolic health
- Regulates blood sugar, lipid profiles and obesity
- Detox improves insulin sensitivity and digestion

Autoimmune Diseases and Spleen Detox
- Detox supports immune balance
- Reduces autoimmune flares and inflammation

Clinical Case Histories
- Patient 1: Reduced inflamation with 30-day detox
- Patient 2: Improved blood sugar and cholestorol after 14-day detox

Detox and Inflammation Control
- Detox helps reduce systemic inflammation
- Clears toxin and damaged cells to reduce inflammatory triggers
- Spleen filters blood, reduces inflammation

Overview of Chronic Diseases
- Spleen Qi Dificiency leads to malabsorption and fatigue
- linked to impaired immune and digestive functions
- Spleen's role in blood filtration and immune regulation

Chapter 17: Spleen Detox for Cardiovascular Health

Spleen and Blood Circulation: Strengthening Blood Vessels and Circulation

The spleen's role in **blood circulation** is often overlooked. Still, it is essential for maintaining healthy blood vessels and ensuring that oxygen and nutrients are efficiently delivered to tissues. The spleen filters out **damaged red blood cells** and produces **immune cells** that maintain the integrity of blood vessels. A detox that targets the spleen can help improve blood circulation by removing toxins that contribute to **atherosclerosis** and **high blood pressure**.

In TCM, the spleen and **liver** work together to maintain blood circulation. Detoxing these organs simultaneously can improve overall cardiovascular health, reducing the risk of heart disease.

Analogy: Think of the spleen as a **traffic controller** for blood cells, ensuring that only healthy, functional cells are allowed to circulate. Detoxing the spleen ensures that traffic flows smoothly, reducing the build-up of damaged cells that could clog the system.

IV Therapies and Supplements for Cardiovascular Support (PPC, Glutathione)

Phosphatidylcholine (PPC) and **glutathione** are two powerful compounds that support both spleen and cardiovascular health. **PPC**, a key component of cell membranes, helps repair blood vessel walls and improve circulation. During a detox program, PPC IV therapy can help strengthen blood vessels, reduce **cholesterol levels**, and support the spleen's blood-filtering function.

Glutathione, known as the master antioxidant, reduces oxidative stress and inflammation, two major contributors to cardiovascular disease. By neutralising free radicals, glutathione supports the spleen's ability to filter blood and protect the heart and blood vessels from damage.

Clinical Case History

A 60-year-old man with high blood pressure and early-stage atherosclerosis received glutathione and PPC IV therapy as part of his spleen detox program. After 6 weeks, his blood pressure normalised, and his cholesterol levels improved, illustrating the cardiovascular benefits of detoxification.

Integrating Liver and Spleen Detox for Heart Health

The **liver** and **spleen** are intricately connected in both Western and TCM perspectives, particularly in their roles in blood detoxification and circulation. A comprehensive detox program that targets both organs can improve cardiovascular health by ensuring that toxins and damaged cells are efficiently removed from the bloodstream.

The liver is responsible for processing **toxins** and **fats**. At the same time, the spleen focuses on filtering **blood** and regulating the immune response. When these organs are detoxified together, they work synergistically to reduce **cholesterol**, improve **blood flow**, and protect the heart from inflammation and oxidative damage.

Analogy: Think of the liver and spleen as **partners in a clean-up crew**. The liver processes the waste, while the spleen ensures that only clean, healthy blood circulates. Detoxing both organs ensures the system functions efficiently, keeping the heart and blood vessels healthy.

Summary: Spleen Detox for Cardiovascular Health

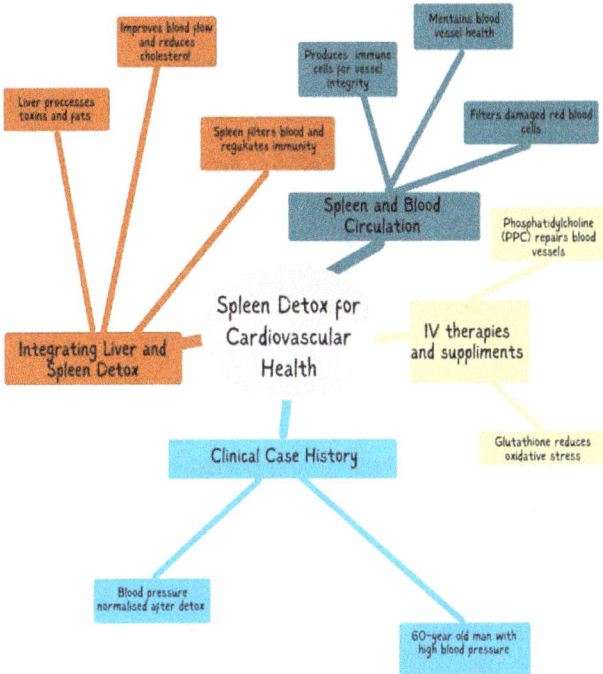

Improves blood flow and reduces cholesterol

Produces immune cells for vessel integrity

Mentains blood vessel health

Liver processes toxins and fats

Spleen filters blood and regulates immunity

Filters damaged red blood cells

Spleen and Blood Circulation

Phosphatidylcholine (PPC) repairs blood vessels

Spleen Detox for Cardiovascular Health

IV therapies and suppliments

Integrating Liver and Spleen Detox

Clinical Case History

Glutathione reduces oxidative stress

Blood pressure normalised after detox

60-year old man with high blood pressure

Chapter 18: Spleen Detox for Gut Health

The Gut-Spleen Connection: Improving Digestion, Bloating, and Leaky Gut

The spleen is closely linked to **digestive health**. In TCM, the spleen is responsible for transforming food into **Qi** and distributing nutrients throughout the body. When the spleen is overburdened by toxins, its ability to digest and absorb nutrients becomes compromised, leading to symptoms like **bloating**, **gas**, and **leaky gut**.

Leaky gut occurs when the intestinal lining becomes damaged, allowing toxins and undigested food particles to enter the bloodstream. A weakened spleen struggles to filter these toxins from the blood, further exacerbating digestive issues and inflammation. A spleen detox can help **repair the gut lining**, reduce inflammation, and improve nutrient absorption.

Clinical Case History

A 42-year-old woman with leaky gut syndrome experienced significant improvements in digestion and energy levels after completing a spleen detox program that included gut-healing foods like bone broth, probiotics, and spleen-supportive herbs like Bai Zhu.

Healing the Gut with Spleen-Focused Diets and Detox Protocols

A spleen-focused diet during detox prioritises easily digestible, warming foods that reduce inflammation and support the digestive system. **Cooked vegetables**, **broths**, **whole grains**, and **probiotics** can help repair the gut lining and reduce digestive symptoms like bloating and gas. Eliminating **sugar**, **processed foods**, and **dairy** from the diet reduces the toxic load on the spleen and gut, promoting better digestion.

Incorporating gut-healing supplements such as **collagen, L-glutamine**, and **digestive enzymes** can also support gut repair during detox. These supplements help restore the integrity of the gut lining and improve nutrient absorption, making it easier for the spleen to transform food into energy.

Analogy: Think of the spleen as the **cook** in your digestive system. A detox gives the cook a break by providing simple, easy-to-digest meals, allowing them to function at their best.

The Role of Probiotics and Digestive Enzymes in Spleen Health

Probiotics and **digestive enzymes** are essential for gut health and play a critical role in supporting spleen function. Probiotics help maintain a healthy balance of **gut bacteria**, which is necessary for proper digestion and immune function. A healthy gut microbiome reduces the burden on the spleen by improving nutrient absorption and reducing inflammation.

Digestive enzymes assist the spleen by breaking down food more effectively, ensuring that nutrients are properly absorbed. Enzyme supplementation during a spleen detox can help ease the digestive burden on the spleen, allowing it to focus on its role in detoxification and immune regulation.

Clinical Case History

A 48-year-old man with chronic bloating and indigestion found relief after incorporating a daily probiotic and digestive enzyme supplement into his spleen detox program. His digestion improved, and he experienced less bloating and discomfort.

Conclusion of Part 6

This section explored the role of spleen detox in managing chronic diseases like **autoimmune disorders**, **metabolic syndrome**, and **cardiovascular disease**. By supporting the spleen through detox programs, individuals can reduce inflammation, improve digestion, and balance immune function, all of which are crucial for managing chronic conditions.

Summary: Spleen Detox for Gut Health

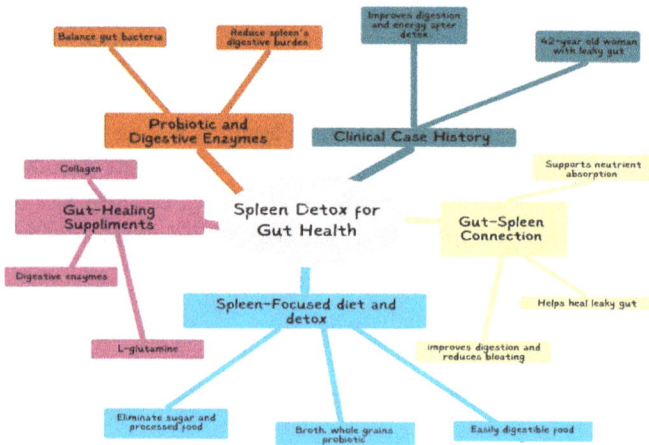

Part 7:
Advanced Detox Techniques—Light Therapy and Endolaser

Chapter 19: Endolaser Light Therapy and Spleen Health

Introduction to Endolaser Therapy: How Light Therapy Works at the Cellular Level

Endolaser light therapy is an innovative treatment that uses **low-level laser light** to stimulate cellular function and improve the body's ability to heal and detoxify. This therapy, also known as **photobiomodulation**, delivers specific wavelengths of light into the body's tissues, which helps stimulate cellular repair, reduce inflammation, and enhance blood circulation. These processes are particularly important for the spleen, as they help to **improve its ability to filter toxins** from the blood and support immune function.

At the cellular level, light therapy works by stimulating **mitochondria**, the energy-producing components of cells. When mitochondria absorb light, they produce more **adenosine triphosphate (ATP)**, the energy currency of cells. This increased energy allows cells to repair damage more quickly, detoxify more effectively, and improve overall function. Light therapy also reduces oxidative stress, which is critical during detox, as it helps protect cells from the damage caused by toxins and inflammation.

Analogy: Think of light therapy as a **recharge station** for your cells. It provides the energy boost they need to detox and repair more efficiently, helping the spleen function at its best.

The Weber Device: Using Endolaser Therapy for Detox

The **Weber Endolaser device** is a specific tool used in advanced detox programs to deliver targeted laser therapy into the body. The Weber device combines different wavelengths of light (red, blue, green, yellow, and infrared) to address various cellular functions.

Each wavelength penetrates tissues at different depths, allowing for precise stimulation of the spleen and other organs involved in detoxification.

For spleen detox, the Weber device can be particularly effective in improving blood flow, reducing inflammation, and enhancing the spleen's immune-regulating functions. By using **intravenous laser therapy**, light can be delivered directly into the bloodstream, enhancing the detoxification process by **stimulating immune cells** and increasing circulation.

Incorporating this therapy into a spleen detox program can result in quicker **toxin removal**, better **immune function**, and an overall improvement in energy levels and well-being. It is especially beneficial for individuals with chronic illnesses or those undergoing intense detoxification programs.

Clinical Case History

A 50-year-old man with chronic fatigue and liver inflammation underwent a 6-week detox that included Weber light therapy. After completing the program, his liver enzymes normalised, and his energy levels improved, highlighting the impact of light therapy on detox processes.

Mechanism of Action: Improving Microcirculation, Cellular Repair, and Detoxification

Endolaser light therapy works by improving **microcirculation**, which is crucial for delivering oxygen and nutrients to cells and removing toxins. Better circulation supports the spleen's role in filtering blood and regulating immune responses. Additionally, by stimulating cellular repair mechanisms and reducing oxidative stress, light therapy helps cells recover from damage caused by toxins and chronic inflammation. This enhances the body's overall ability to detoxify, particularly during a spleen-focused detox program.

Summary: Endolaser Light Therapy and Spleen Health

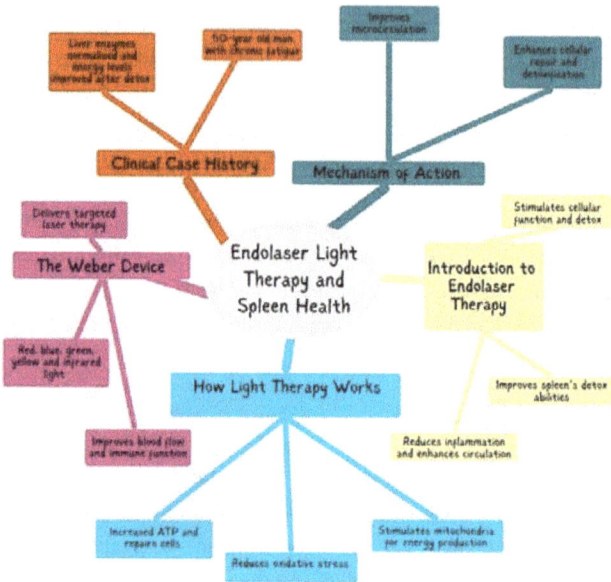

Mind map: Endolaser Light Therapy and Spleen Health

- Clinical Case History
  - Liver enzymes normalized and energy levels improved after detox
  - 50-year-old man with chronic fatigue
- Mechanism of Action
  - Improves microcirculation
  - Enhances cellular repair and detoxification
- The Weber Device
  - Delivers targeted laser therapy
  - Red, blue, green, yellow and infrared light
  - Improves blood flow and immune function
- Introduction to Endolaser Therapy
  - Stimulates cellular function and detox
  - Improves spleen's detox abilities
  - Reduces inflammation and enhances circulation
- How Light Therapy Works
  - Increased ATP and repairs cells
  - Reduces oxidative stress
  - Stimulates mitochondria for energy production

Chapter 20: Benefits of Endolaser Light Therapy in Spleen Detox

Reducing Inflammation with Light Therapy

Chronic **inflammation** is a common issue in individuals with **Spleen Qi Deficiency** or those undergoing detox for chronic diseases. Inflammation can overwhelm the spleen, impairing its ability to filter toxins from the blood and regulate immune function. Endolaser light therapy can reduce inflammation at the cellular level by modulating the body's production of **pro-inflammatory cytokines** and stimulating the release of **anti-inflammatory mediators**.

Light therapy has been shown to lower levels of **C-reactive protein (CRP)**, an important marker of systemic inflammation. By reducing these levels, the spleen can work more efficiently, allowing the body to detoxify more effectively. This is particularly useful for individuals with chronic conditions like **arthritis, autoimmune diseases**, or **metabolic syndrome**, where inflammation plays a significant role in disease progression.

Clinical Case History

A 55-year-old woman with rheumatoid arthritis reported reduced joint pain and inflammation after incorporating Endolaser therapy into her detox program. Inflammation markers, including CRP, dropped significantly, showing how light therapy can reduce inflammation and support spleen health.

Boosting Immune Function and Spleen Qi

The spleen is a key organ in regulating the body's **immune system**, and detoxification can be particularly taxing on the immune system, especially if the body is dealing with a large toxic load. **Endolaser therapy** can help **boost immune function** by stimulating the production of **white blood cells** and improving the activity of **macrophages**, which are responsible for engulfing and destroying pathogens and toxins in the bloodstream.

By improving **Spleen Qi**, or the energy the spleen uses to transform food into nutrients and energy, Endolaser therapy helps support the spleen's digestive and immune functions. A spleen detox that incorporates light therapy is not only removing toxins but also **re-energising** the spleen's natural ability to maintain balance in the body.

Analogy: Think of the immune system as an army defending your body from invaders. Endolaser light therapy strengthens the army's numbers. It equips it with better tools to fight off pathogens, ensuring that the spleen can focus on detoxifying the blood and maintaining overall balance.

Enhancing Cellular Energy and Detox Pathways

By stimulating the production of **ATP** and enhancing **mitochondrial function**, Endolaser therapy provides a significant boost to cellular energy levels. This is crucial during detoxification, as detox pathways like the liver and spleen require a great deal of energy to process and eliminate toxins. Light therapy helps improve the efficiency of these detox pathways by ensuring that cells have the energy they need to perform their functions optimally.

Summary: Benefits of Endolaser Light Therapy in Spleen Detox

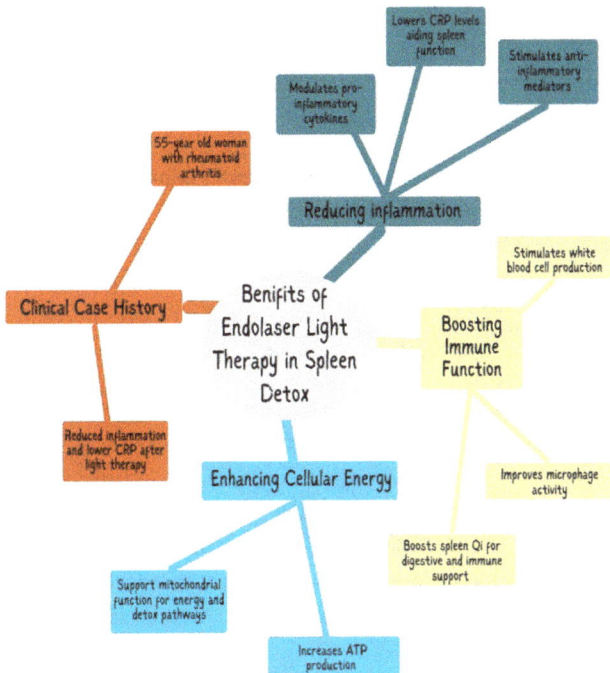

Benifits of Endolaser Light Therapy in Spleen Detox

Reducing inflammation
- Lowers CRP levels aiding spleen function
- Stimulates anti-inflammatory mediators
- Modulates pro-inflammatory cytokines

Clinical Case History
- 55-year old woman with rheumatoid arthritis
- Reduced inflammation and lower CRP after light therapy

Boosting Immune Function
- Stimulates white blood cell production
- Improves microphage activity
- Boosts spleen Qi for digestive and immune support

Enhancing Cellular Energy
- Support mitochondrial function for energy and detox pathways
- Increases ATP production

Chapter 21: Integrating Light Therapy with Other Detox Methods

Combining Endolaser Therapy with IV Drips for Optimal Results

For individuals undergoing a spleen detox, combining **Endolaser light therapy** with **IV nutrient drips** can dramatically improve the detox process. IV therapy delivers essential nutrients, vitamins, and antioxidants directly into the bloodstream, supporting detoxification. In contrast, light therapy stimulates **cellular repair** and improves circulation. Together, these therapies create a synergistic effect, allowing the body to process and eliminate toxins more efficiently.

For example, pairing IV **glutathione** or **vitamin C** with light therapy can enhance the body's ability to fight oxidative stress and improve the spleen's blood-filtering capabilities. This approach is particularly useful for individuals with **chronic fatigue**, **autoimmune disorders**, or **inflammatory diseases**, where both immune function and detox pathways are compromised.

Clinical Case History

A 45-year-old woman with chronic Lyme disease combined IV vitamin C with Endolaser light therapy during a detox program. She reported improved energy levels, reduced brain fog, and a significant reduction in inflammation markers, demonstrating the effectiveness of combining these therapies for detoxification.

Scheduling Treatments for Maximum Spleen Detox Benefits

To achieve the best results, Endolaser light therapy should be scheduled **1-2 times per week** during a spleen detox program.

Depending on the individual's health status, light therapy may be paired with other treatments like **IV drips**, **fasting**, or **herbal supplementation**. A well-rounded detox program that integrates these therapies can help optimise the body's natural detoxification pathways and support the spleen's function in blood filtration and immune regulation.

For individuals with more severe conditions, like **autoimmune diseases** or **chronic inflammatory conditions**, it may be beneficial to increase the frequency of treatments during the initial stages of the detox. Over time, treatments can be tapered down as the body begins to heal and detoxify more efficiently.

Analogy: Think of detox like a **thorough house cleaning**. Just as you wouldn't rush through deep cleaning in one day, spreading out treatments over several weeks ensures that each aspect of the detox is fully addressed without overwhelming the body.

Case Studies: Using Light Therapy in Chronic Disease Management and Detox

Case Study 1: A 60-year-old man with metabolic syndrome, high cholesterol, and poor circulation incorporated Endolaser therapy into his 8-week detox program. After completing the program, his cholesterol levels improved, circulation increased, and he reported a significant reduction in joint inflammation.

Case Study 2: A 38-year-old woman with lupus and chronic fatigue integrated light therapy into her detox plan, resulting in fewer autoimmune flare-ups, improved energy levels, and better overall well-being.

These cases highlight the effectiveness of combining Endolaser therapy with detox strategies for managing chronic diseases and supporting spleen health.

Conclusion of Part 7

Part 7 has explored the advanced detox techniques of **Endolaser light therapy** and its role in supporting spleen health. By improving circulation, reducing inflammation, and enhancing immune function, light therapy plays a crucial role in optimising detox programs and supporting individuals with chronic health conditions. When combined with other therapies, like **IV drips**, it creates a powerful detoxification strategy that promotes overall well-being and restores balance to the body.

Summary: Integrating Light Therapy with Other Detox Methods

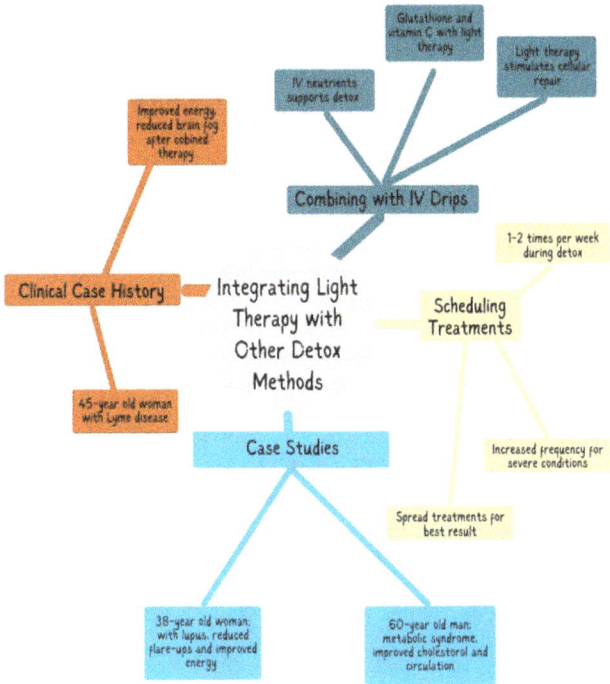

Glatathione and vitamin C with light therapy

Light therapy stimulates cellular repair

IV neutrients supports detox

Improved energy, reduced brain fog after cobined therapy

Combining with IV Drips

Clinical Case History

Integrating Light Therapy with Other Detox Methods

1-2 times per week during detox

Scheduling Treatments

45-year old woman with Lyme disease

Case Studies

Increased frequency for severe conditions

Spread treatments for best result

38-year old woman, with lupus, reduced flare-ups and improved energy

60-year old man, metabolic syndrome, improved cholestorol and circulation

Part 8:
Ancient History of Spleen Detox

Chapter 22: Spleen Detoxification in Ancient Civilisations

Ancient Egypt: The Understanding of the Spleen in Early Medicine

In **Ancient Egypt**, the spleen was seen as an essential organ for both physical and spiritual health. Egyptian medical texts like the **Ebers Papyrus**, dating back to around 1550 BCE, mention the spleen in connection to blood disorders and immune function. However, they did not fully understand its exact role. The Egyptians used herbal remedies, such as **garlic** and **onions**, which were believed to purify the blood and aid in the detoxification of the spleen.

They also associated the spleen with the **afterlife**, as it was one of the organs removed and preserved during the mummification process. This indicates that the Egyptians believed in the spleen's importance beyond mere physical health, linking it to **spiritual well-being**. While their anatomical understanding was limited, they clearly valued the spleen as an essential organ, using herbs and **natural detoxification methods** to support its function.

Analogy: Think of the ancient Egyptians as early practitioners of holistic health, recognising that organs like the spleen played both physical and spiritual roles in the body's overall wellness.

Ancient Greece: Hippocrates' View on Spleen Health and Detoxification

The **ancient Greeks**, particularly the physician **Hippocrates**, also recognised the importance of the spleen in maintaining overall health. Hippocrates, often called the "father of modern medicine," believed that the spleen was involved in the body's **balance of** humor—a concept central to Greek medicine. The humors were thought to be bodily fluids that needed to be balanced for a person to remain healthy. An excess of **black bile**, which was believed to be processed by the spleen, could result in diseases such as **melancholy** (depression) and **digestive disorders**.

To promote spleen health and balance the humors, the ancient Greeks recommended dietary changes and herbal treatments. Foods that were easy to digest, such as **grains**, **honey**, and **fruits**, were emphasised, and bitter herbs like **wormwood** were used to stimulate digestion and detoxify the spleen.

In ancient Greek medicine, maintaining spleen health was seen as essential to keeping the body's overall balance and preventing disease. However, their understanding of its physiological function was more symbolic than scientific.

Clinical Case History (Hypothetical):

A patient presenting with depressive symptoms and digestive issues might have been diagnosed with an imbalance of black bile by Hippocrates and treated with herbs and dietary changes to restore spleen function.

Traditional Chinese Medicine: The Spleen as the Centre of Digestion and Energy

In **Traditional Chinese Medicine (TCM)**, the spleen plays a central role in both **digestion** and **energy production**. The spleen is responsible for transforming food into **Qi**, the body's life force, and distributing this energy throughout the body. Unlike the Western view, which often sees the spleen as secondary to organs like the liver or stomach, TCM views the spleen as foundational to overall health.

In TCM, an imbalance in the spleen is believed to lead to conditions such as **bloating**, **fatigue**, and **poor appetite**. The ancient Chinese developed a comprehensive approach to spleen health that included a balanced diet, **herbal remedies**, and lifestyle practices like **Qi Gong** to strengthen the spleen's function.

Foods that are **warm** and **nourishing**—such as **cooked grains**, **root vegetables**, and **warming spices** like ginger—are recommended to support spleen health. The belief is that cold or raw foods weaken the spleen's energy, making it less effective at digesting food and transforming nutrients into energy.

Clinical Case History:

A 45-year-old woman experiencing chronic fatigue and bloating would be diagnosed with **Spleen Qi Deficiency** in TCM. Her treatment might include warm soups, cooked grains, and herbal tonics like **Dang Shen** and **Bai Zhu** to restore balance.

Ayurveda: The Role of the Spleen in Balancing Doshas

In **Ayurvedic medicine**, the spleen is closely linked to the **Pitta Dosha**, which governs metabolism, digestion, and the body's ability to transform and process food. The spleen is considered part of the **Rasa Dhatu**, or the body's circulatory system of fluids. When the spleen becomes overloaded with toxins, it disrupts the Pitta Dosha, leading to conditions such as **inflammation, indigestion**, and **low energy**.

Ayurveda recommends a **detoxification process** known as **Panchakarma** to cleanse and restore balance to the spleen and other digestive organs. Panchakarma involves a combination of **oil massages, herbal treatments**, and **cleansing techniques** like **basti (enemas)** and **virechana (purgation)** to remove toxins and balance the doshas.

Essential Ayurvedic herbs like **Guduchi, Triphala**, and **Neem** are often used to support the spleen's detoxification processes and help balance the body's energy levels. These herbs are believed to cleanse the blood, reduce inflammation, and support the digestive system.

Clinical Case History:

A 50-year-old man with symptoms of indigestion and sluggish digestion would undergo a Panchakarma detox in Ayurveda, using herbs like Triphala and Guduchi to purify the blood and restore spleen function.

Summary: Spleen Detoxification in Ancient Civilisations

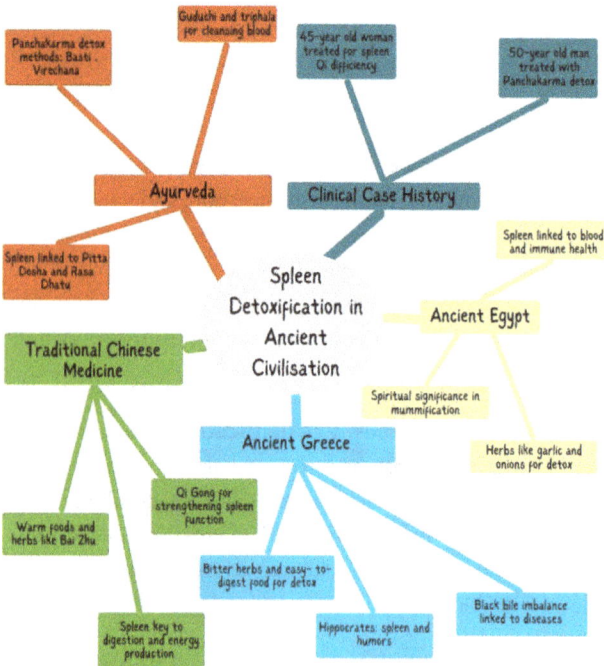

Chapter 23: Spleen Detox in Ayurveda

Ayurveda's Perspective on the Spleen: The Importance of Rasa and Rakta Dhatus

In Ayurveda, the spleen is part of the **Rasa Dhatu** and **Rakta Dhatu**, two of the body's seven tissues responsible for nourishing the body and maintaining its vitality. The Rasa Dhatu is the primary nourishing fluid that supports the formation of blood. At the same time, the Rakta Dhatu is associated with the circulatory system, providing nourishment to muscles and tissues. The spleen plays a key role in filtering these fluids and maintaining their purity, thus supporting the body's overall vitality.

When the spleen becomes overloaded with **Ama** (toxins), it can disrupt the balance of these dhatus, leading to conditions like **poor digestion, anaemia, chronic fatigue**, and **immune dysfunction**. Ayurveda focuses on removing **Ama** through detoxification practices to restore balance to the Rasa and Rakta Dhatus and support spleen health.

The concept of **Agni**, or digestive fire, is also closely linked to spleen health in Ayurveda. A strong Agni ensures that food is properly digested and transformed into Rasa. At the same time, a weak Agni leads to the accumulation of toxins. Maintaining spleen health is essential for keeping Agni strong and promoting overall well-being.

Spleen and the Doshas: Balancing Pitta for Optimal Spleen Health

The spleen is most closely associated with the **Pitta Dosha**, which governs **digestion**, **metabolism**, and **transformation** in the body. When the Pitta Dosha is out of balance, it can lead to excessive heat, inflammation, and digestive issues. This imbalance can overload the spleen, causing it to become sluggish and unable to effectively filter toxins from the blood.

Ayurvedic practices for balancing Pitta often focus on **cooling** the body and reducing inflammation. Foods like **cucumbers, melons**, and **leafy greens** are emphasised, while **spicy, oily**, and **fried foods** are avoided, as they can exacerbate Pitta imbalance.

Herbs like **Guduchi** and **Amla** are also used to cool the body and reduce Pitta-related inflammation, supporting spleen function by reducing the burden of excess heat and toxins. Lifestyle practices like **meditation, yoga**, and **oil massages** with cooling oils (such as **coconut oil**) are also recommended to help balance Pitta and support spleen health.

Analogy: Think of the Pitta Dosha as a **fire**. If the fire becomes too strong, it can burn out the spleen's ability to function effectively. Cooling herbs and foods help keep the fire at a manageable level, allowing the spleen to detox and filter the blood properly.

Ayurvedic Detox Practices: Panchakarma, Rasayana, and Herbal Remedies for Spleen Health

Ayurveda's **Panchakarma** detox practice is one of the most comprehensive approaches to cleansing the body and restoring spleen health. Panchakarma consists of five cleansing techniques: **Vamana** (therapeutic vomiting), **Virechana** (purgation), **Basti** (enemas), **Nasya** (nasal treatments), and **Raktamokshana** (bloodletting). These techniques are used to eliminate toxins from the body, balance the doshas, and improve the spleen's ability to filter and cleanse the blood.

Alongside Panchakarma, **Rasayana** therapies focus on rejuvenating the body's tissues and strengthening the spleen. **Herbs** like **Ashwagandha, Shatavari**, and **Brahmi** are commonly used to rebuild vitality and support the digestive system after detoxification.

Triphala, a combination of three fruits (Amalaki, Bibhitaki, and Haritaki), is one of the most widely used herbal remedies in Ayurveda for spleen health. It acts as a gentle detoxifier, helping to cleanse the digestive system and support the spleen's role in blood filtration.

Clinical Case History:

A 35-year-old woman experiencing digestive disturbances and low energy underwent a Panchakarma detox focused on spleen health, followed by Rasayana therapies. After completing the program, she reported improved digestion, clearer skin, and increased vitality.

Key Ayurvedic Herbs: Triphala, Guduchi, and Neem for Spleen Function

Ayurveda places a strong emphasis on herbal remedies to support spleen function and detoxification. Some of the most important herbs for spleen health include:

- **Triphala**: A blend of three fruits, Triphala is a gentle yet powerful detoxifier that supports the digestive system and helps cleanse the spleen of toxins. It is often used to promote healthy bowel movements and improve nutrient absorption.

- **Guduchi**: Known as the "nectar of immortality," Guduchi is a potent anti-inflammatory herb that helps cool excess Pitta, supports the immune system, and improves the spleen's ability to filter toxins from the blood.

- **Neem**: This bitter herb is known for its purifying properties, particularly in relation to blood detoxification. Neem helps cleanse the spleen and liver, promoting healthy circulation and immune function.

These herbs can be used in **teas**, **powders**, or **capsules** as part of a comprehensive spleen detox program, helping to reduce inflammation, improve digestion, and support the spleen's natural detoxification processes.

Conclusion of Part 8

This section has explored the role of the spleen in ancient medical systems, including **Ancient Egypt**, **Ancient Greece**, **Traditional Chinese Medicine**, and **Ayurveda**. Each of these systems recognised the importance of spleen health and developed detoxification techniques and herbal remedies to support its function. By integrating ancient wisdom with modern detox practices, we can develop a holistic approach to spleen health that incorporates both physical and emotional well-being.

Summary: Spleen Detox in Ayurveda

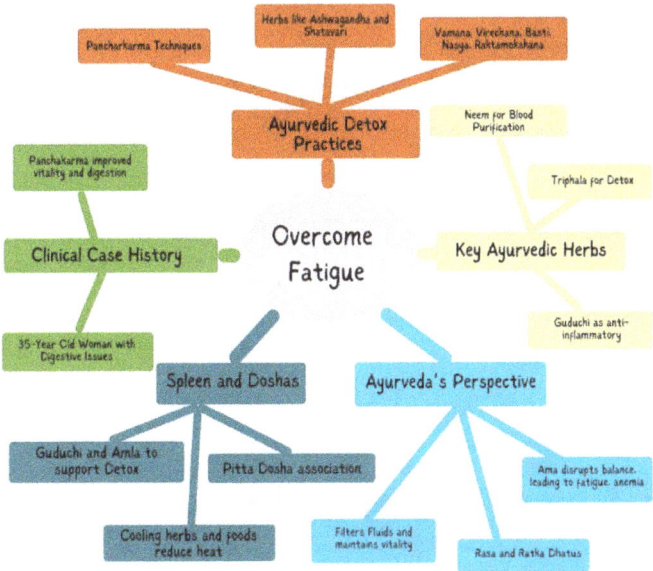

Part 9:
Long-Term Spleen Health

Chapter 24: Maintaining Spleen Health After Detox

Daily Routines for Optimal Spleen Function

Maintaining long-term spleen health requires adopting daily habits that support the organ's function and reduce the risk of toxin build-up. After completing a detox, it is important to continue practices that strengthen the spleen's ability to regulate **digestion, energy production**, and **immune function**.

A **daily routine** for spleen health should include:

1. **Warming, Nourishing Foods**: As highlighted in **Traditional Chinese Medicine (TCM)**, consuming **warm, cooked foods** helps protect and nourish the spleen. Avoid raw, cold foods and excess sugar, which can weaken the spleen's energy. Instead, focus on meals rich in **root vegetables, whole grains**, and **soups** that are easy to digest and support the spleen's function.

2. **Hydration**: Drinking warm or room-temperature water throughout the day helps maintain digestive health and assists the spleen in transporting nutrients throughout the body. Adding **ginger** or **lemon** to water can further support digestion and circulation.

3. **Rest and Recovery**: Ensure you get **adequate sleep** each night (7-9 hours), as rest is critical for spleen health. During sleep, the body repairs itself and eliminates toxins. A regular sleep routine helps support the spleen's role in maintaining immune and digestive functions.

4. **Moderate Exercise**: Gentle exercises such as **walking, Qi Gong**, and **yoga** promote circulation and stimulate the lymphatic system, aiding the spleen in filtering blood and removing toxins. Strenuous exercise, which can weaken

the spleen in some cases, should be avoided in favour of moderate, regular movement.

Analogy: Think of your spleen as a **garden**. Just as a garden needs consistent watering, nourishing soil, and occasional pruning, your spleen thrives when given proper care, gentle movement, and nutrient-rich food on a daily basis.

Long-Term Nutritional Practices

The spleen's role in digestion and nutrient absorption makes **long-term dietary habits** key to maintaining its health. Beyond detox, incorporating specific **spleen-friendly foods** into your everyday meals can ensure that your spleen remains strong and efficient.

Critical nutritional practices for spleen health include:

- **Cooked, Easy-to-Digest Foods**: Foods like **brown rice**, **quinoa**, and **steamed vegetables** are easy on the digestive system and help support the spleen's function. Cooking breaks down the fibres in food, making it easier for the body to absorb nutrients without placing too much strain on the spleen.

- **Healthy Fats**: Incorporate healthy fats such as **avocado**, **olive oil**, and **coconut oil** into your diet. These fats provide essential nutrients without burdening the spleen, unlike processed or fried foods.

- **Warming Spices**: Use spices like **ginger**, **turmeric**, **cinnamon**, and **cardamom** to support digestion and circulation. These spices help stimulate the spleen's Qi and improve nutrient absorption.

- **Probiotic-Rich Foods**: Incorporate foods like **yoghurt**, **sauerkraut**, **kimchi**, and **miso** to support gut health and immune function. A healthy gut microbiome enhances the spleen's ability to filter blood and manage toxins.

In the long term, avoiding foods that create **dampness** in the body, such as dairy, excess sugar, and processed grains, is essential to maintaining spleen health. These foods can overwhelm the spleen, leading to symptoms like bloating, fatigue, and weight gain.

Clinical Case History

A 42-year-old man with digestive issues and frequent fatigue switched to a spleen-friendly diet of warm, cooked meals with healthy fats and spices. After three months, his energy levels increased, and his digestion improved, showing the long-term benefits of adopting a spleen-supportive diet.

Preventing Spleen Qi Deficiency

Spleen Qi Deficiency is a common diagnosis in TCM, characterised by symptoms such as **fatigue**, **poor digestion**, **bloating**, and **weak immunity**. To prevent this deficiency from occurring or recurring after a detox, it is vital to maintain habits that promote spleen health and prevent the build-up of toxins or excess stress on the spleen.

Critical practices for preventing Spleen Qi Deficiency include:

- **Managing Stress**: Chronic stress can weaken the spleen's ability to transform food into energy. Practices such as **meditation**, **deep breathing**, and **mindfulness** help manage stress levels, preventing the spleen from becoming overburdened.

- **Eating Regular, Balanced Meals**: Skipping meals or eating irregularly weakens the spleen, as it thrives on routine. Make it a habit to eat small, balanced meals at regular intervals to support digestion and energy production. Avoid overeating, as this can also strain the spleen.

- **Avoiding Excessive Cold**: Both environmental cold (like cold weather) and cold foods can damage spleen function. Dress warmly in cold climates and focus on warm, cooked meals rather than cold salads or raw fruits and vegetables.

- **Herbal Support**: Herbs like **Astragalus** (Huang Qi), **Ginseng**, and **Liquorice Root** can help strengthen the spleen and boost energy levels. These herbs can be taken as teas, powders, or supplements and are often included in long-term health maintenance plans.

Analogy: Think of Spleen Qi as the **fuel** that keeps your body running smoothly. If the spleen is overworked or undernourished, it runs low on fuel, making it difficult to maintain optimal health.

Summary: Maintaining Spleen Health After Detox

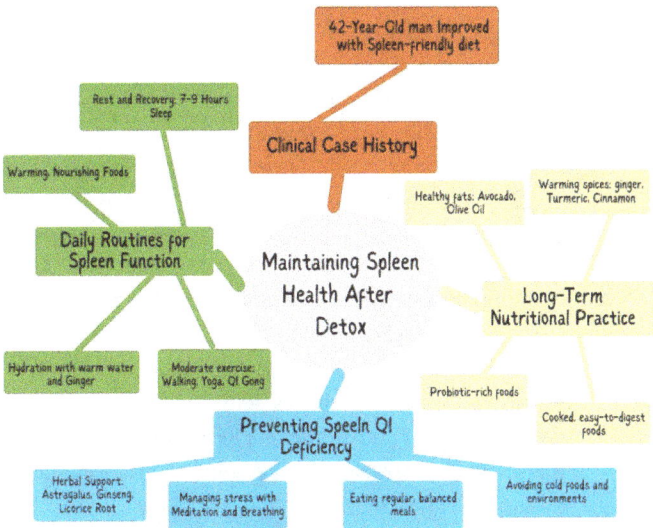

Mind map: Maintaining Spleen Health After Detox

- 42-Year-Old man Improved with Spleen-friendly diet
- Clinical Case History
- Rest and Recovery: 7-9 Hours Sleep
- Warming, Nourishing Foods
- Daily Routines for Spleen Function
- Hydration with warm water and Ginger
- Moderate exercise: Walking, Yoga, QI Gong
- Healthy fats: Avocado, Olive Oil
- Warming spices: ginger, Turmeric, Cinnamon
- Long-Term Nutritional Practice
- Probiotic-rich foods
- Cooked, easy-to-digest foods
- Preventing Speeln QI Deficiency
- Herbal Support: Astragalus, Ginseng, Licorice Root
- Managing stress with Meditation and Breathing
- Eating regular, balanced meals
- Avoiding cold foods and environments

Chapter 25: Seasonal Cleansing Throughout the Year

How to Adjust Your Detox for Each Season

Different seasons affect the body's organs in various ways, and **seasonal cleansing** helps ensure that the spleen and other organs stay in balance year-round. In TCM, each season corresponds to different organs, and adjusting your detox practices to align with these natural rhythms can support long-term health.

- **Spring (Liver and Spleen Focus)**: Spring is the ideal time for a spleen detox, as the body naturally shifts toward renewal and growth. During spring, focus on **light, fresh foods** like green vegetables and cleansing herbs (e.g., **dandelion root** and **nettles**). These foods help detoxify the liver and spleen, clearing out toxins accumulated during the winter months.

- **Summer (Heart and Small Intestine Focus)**: Summer corresponds to the **heart** and **small intestine** in TCM, which means that a lighter detox focused on hydration and cooling foods is beneficial. Incorporate **cucumber, watermelon,** and **mint** into your diet to cool and cleanse the body. Though the spleen benefits from lighter foods, avoid too many cold or raw foods, which could weaken spleen Qi.

- **Autumn (Lung and Large Intestine Focus)**: As the weather cools, focus on **nourishing, grounding foods** that support the **lungs** and **large intestine** while maintaining spleen health. Foods like **sweet potatoes, pumpkin,** and **carrots** provide warmth and grounding energy, helping to maintain a balanced digestive system.

- **Winter (Kidney and Bladder Focus)**: Winter is the time to rest and nourish the **kidneys** and **bladder**. During this season, **warming stews**, **broths**, and **hearty grains** help support the spleen while nourishing the kidneys. Avoid cold and raw foods, which can overburden the digestive system. Herbal teas like **ginger**, **cinnamon**, and **turmeric** keep the body warm and the spleen supported throughout the colder months.

Analogy: Just as you might change your wardrobe with the seasons, adjusting your detox practices ensures that your body's organs, including the spleen, are properly supported all year long.

Seasonal Foods and Practices

Spring Detox: During the spring, focus on foods that help clear out stagnation and support spleen health. Leafy greens, asparagus, artichokes, and sprouts are ideal for spring detox, as they promote gentle cleansing and reduce inflammation. Consider incorporating **herbal teas** made with **dandelion**, **milk thistle**, or **burdock root**, which are known for their liver and spleen cleansing properties.

Summer Detox: Summer calls for light, hydrating foods that cool the body. Fresh fruits like watermelon, berries, and citrus help cleanse the body while keeping you hydrated. Focus on **cooling herbs** like **mint** and **cilantro** to balance the heat of the season while still ensuring that the spleen is supported with warm, cooked meals.

Autumn Detox: As the weather cools, your diet should shift to include **root vegetables**, **whole grains**, and warming spices. Pumpkins, squash, and parsnips help ground the body and support digestion. Warming teas with **ginger** or **cinnamon** can also support the spleen and help prevent cold-induced digestive issues.

Winter Detox: Winter detoxes should be gentle, focusing on warming, nourishing foods that support the spleen and kidneys. **Bone broths**, **legumes**, and **whole grains** like quinoa and millet provide the necessary warmth and nourishment for the colder months. Herbal teas made with **cinnamon**, **cardamom**, and **ginger** keep the digestive system strong and supported.

Aligning Your Detox with Nature

Aligning your detox with the seasons means respecting your body's natural rhythms and working with nature to support your health. Each season brings its own challenges and opportunities, and your detox practices should reflect these changes. For example, in the spring, the body is naturally inclined toward renewal, making it the best time for a more intensive detox that focuses on liver and spleen health. In contrast, winter is a time for rest and nourishment, so detox practices should be gentler, focusing on warming, nourishing foods that sustain energy through colder months.

By aligning your detox practices with nature, you help ensure that your body stays in balance throughout the year. This holistic approach can prevent imbalances from occurring, support overall well-being, and promote long-term spleen health.

Analogy: Just as farmers adjust their crops based on the season, you can adjust your detox practices to align with your body's natural cycles, ensuring that your spleen and other organs remain healthy and balanced year-round.

Conclusion of Part 9

This section explored the importance of maintaining long-term spleen health after detox, offering practical advice on daily routines, nutrition, and seasonal detox practices. By adopting these habits, you can support your spleen's ability to filter toxins, regulate digestion, and maintain immune function, ensuring optimal health throughout the year.

Summary: Seasonal Cleansing Throughout the Year

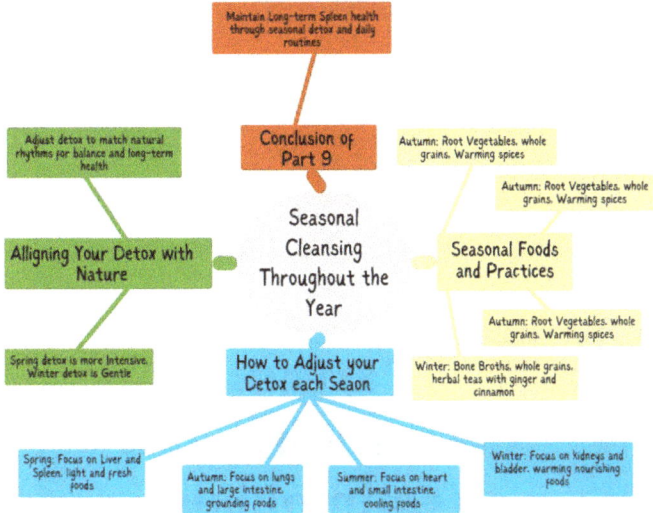

Maintain Long-term Spleen health through seasonal detox and daily routines

Conclusion of Part 9

Adjust detox to match natural rhythms for balance and long-term health

Alligning Your Detox with Nature

Spring detox is more Intensive, Winter detox is Gentle

Seasonal Cleansing Throughout the Year

Autumn: Root Vegetables, whole grains, Warming spices

Autumn: Root Vegetables, whole grains, Warming spices

Seasonal Foods and Practices

Autumn: Root Vegetables, whole grains, Warming spices

Winter: Bone Broths, whole grains, herbal teas with ginger and cinnamon

How to Adjust your Detox each Seaon

Spring: Focus on Liver and Spleen, light and fresh foods

Autumn: Focus on lungs and large intestine, grounding foods

Summer: Focus on heart and small intestine, cooling foods

Winter: Focus on kidneys and bladder, warming nourishing foods

Part 10:
Case Studies and
Testimonials

Chapter 26: Real-Life Spleen Detox Transformations

Case Studies: Before and After

In this section, we will explore multiple real-life examples of individuals who experienced profound changes in their health after completing a spleen detox. These case studies will show how a detoxification program focused on the spleen can improve digestion, energy levels, immune function and help manage chronic conditions.

Case Study 1: Digestive and Energy Improvement in a Middle-Aged Woman

Before:

Emily, 42, had been suffering from chronic **bloating**, **indigestion**, and **low energy** for the past five years. She also had frequent colds and respiratory infections, which left her feeling run down. Despite following various diets and taking supplements, she saw little improvement in her symptoms. Emily's primary complaint was constant bloating after meals, which made her uncomfortable and fatigued throughout the day.

Spleen Detox Protocol:

Emily was placed on a **30-day spleen detox plan** that emphasised **warm, easily digestible foods**, including soups, steamed vegetables, and whole grains like quinoa and millet. She avoided raw or cold foods, as per **Traditional Chinese Medicine (TCM)** principles, to avoid overwhelming the spleen. Her protocol also included daily **herbal teas** with **ginger**, **Bai Zhu**, and **Astragalus** to support digestion and energy production. Gentle Qi Gong exercises were integrated to promote circulation and stimulate spleen function.

After:

By the end of the 30-day detox, Emily reported significant improvements in her digestive health. She no longer experienced bloating after meals, and her energy levels were much higher. Emily also noticed a reduction in the frequency of her colds, indicating an improvement in her immune system. The results encouraged her to maintain some of the dietary and lifestyle practices from the detox, which continued to support her long-term health.

Case Study 2: Autoimmune Disease and Chronic Fatigue

Before:

David, 47, had been diagnosed with **autoimmune thyroiditis** five years earlier. He experienced **chronic fatigue**, **brain fog**, and **joint pain**, making it difficult to manage his day-to-day life. His autoimmune condition often caused flare-ups of inflammation that left him bedridden for days. Conventional treatments helped reduce the severity of his symptoms but did not fully address the root cause of his fatigue and inflammation.

Spleen Detox Protocol:

David underwent a **30-day spleen detox**, which focused on reducing **systemic inflammation** and supporting immune regulation. His detox plan included an **anti-inflammatory diet** rich in vegetables, lean proteins, and anti-inflammatory herbs like **turmeric** and **ginger**. He received weekly **glutathione IV drips** to reduce oxidative stress and improve his energy levels. In addition, David practised **yoga** and **mindfulness meditation** daily to manage his stress and prevent autoimmune flare-ups.

After:

After completing the detox, David reported a dramatic reduction in his fatigue. His energy levels were noticeably higher, and his brain fog lifted, allowing him to focus and work more effectively. He also experienced fewer autoimmune flare-ups, and his joint pain diminished. Blood tests showed reduced levels of inflammation, confirming the benefits of the spleen detox in managing his condition. David continues to follow a modified version of the detox diet and lifestyle practices to maintain these improvements.

Case Study 3: Weight Loss and Blood Sugar Management in a Prediabetic Man

Before:

Jason, 52, had been diagnosed with **prediabetes** and struggled to control his **blood sugar levels**. He was overweight and experienced frequent sugar cravings, bloating, and low energy, which made it difficult for him to lose weight and manage his condition. His doctor had recommended a low-sugar diet, but Jason found it difficult to stick to these dietary changes and often felt sluggish.

Spleen Detox Protocol:

Jason followed a **14-day spleen detox** with a focus on balancing blood sugar and reducing inflammation. His plan included **low-glycaemic foods** such as leafy greens, quinoa, and bitter melon to help regulate his blood sugar. Jason was also prescribed **herbal teas** with **berberine** and **bitter herbs** to reduce sugar cravings and improve digestion. He practised daily walking and gentle yoga to stimulate circulation and support spleen function. Jason received **vitamin C IV therapy** twice during the detox to boost his immune system and reduce oxidative stress.

After:

At the end of the 14-day detox, Jason had lost 8 pounds, and his **fasting blood sugar levels** had improved significantly. He reported feeling more energetic, with reduced sugar cravings and improved digestion. His doctor was pleased with his progress, and Jason continued to follow the low-glycaemic diet and gentle exercise plan after the detox, which helped him maintain his weight loss and manage his prediabetes more effectively.

Case Study 4: Reducing IBS Symptoms with a Spleen Detox

Before:

Sophia, 36, had been suffering from **Irritable Bowel Syndrome (IBS)** for several years. Her symptoms included **bloating**, **constipation**, and **abdominal pain** after meals. Sophia also experienced frequent anxiety, which exacerbated her digestive issues. Her condition was impacting her quality of life, and she was eager to find a natural solution to her IBS symptoms.

Spleen Detox Protocol:

Sophia embarked on a **21-day spleen detox** focused on calming her digestive system and reducing inflammation. She followed a diet of **cooked vegetables, whole grains,** and **spleen-friendly herbs** such as **Triphala** and **fennel**. She also incorporated **probiotic-rich foods** like **sauerkraut** and **yoghurt** to restore gut balance. To manage her anxiety, Sophia practised **mindfulness meditation** and **deep breathing exercises** daily.

After:

By the end of the 21-day detox, Sophia's IBS symptoms had improved significantly. Her bloating was reduced, she experienced regular bowel movements, and her abdominal pain decreased. She also felt more relaxed and in control of her anxiety, which further supported her digestive health. Sophia continued to use the diet and stress management techniques she learned during the detox to maintain her improved digestion and well-being.

Expert Opinions and Insights

Experts in **Traditional Chinese Medicine (TCM)** and **Western integrative medicine** provide valuable insights into the role of spleen detox in promoting overall health and managing chronic conditions.

Spleen Clean

Dr Mei Li, a TCM practitioner and acupuncturist, emphasises the spleen's vital role in digestion and energy:

"In TCM, the spleen is the foundation of digestion and energy production. When the spleen becomes weak, we see symptoms like bloating, fatigue, and immune issues. A well-planned spleen detox helps strengthen Spleen Qi, improve nutrient absorption, and boost immunity. By nourishing the spleen with warm, cooked foods and incorporating spleen-strengthening herbs, we can restore balance to the body."

– Dr Mei Li

Dr Andrew Green, an integrative medicine specialist, explains the impact of detoxing the spleen on chronic inflammation:

"In Western medicine, we often overlook the spleen's role in managing inflammation. By filtering damaged cells and toxins from the blood, the spleen plays a key role in immune regulation. For patients dealing with chronic inflammation, detoxing the spleen can help reduce the overall inflammatory burden and improve immune function. I often recommend combining a spleen detox with IV antioxidant therapies, such as glutathione or vitamin C, to accelerate the detox process."

– Dr Andrew Green

Dr Priya Gupta, an Ayurvedic practitioner, highlights the importance of detoxing the spleen to balance the body's doshas, particularly **Pitta**:

"In Ayurveda, the spleen is connected to the Pitta dosha, which governs digestion and transformation in the body. When toxins accumulate, Pitta becomes imbalanced, leading to inflammation and digestive issues. A spleen detox using herbs like Triphala and Guduchi, along with practices like yoga and meditation, can help cool Pitta and restore digestive balance. Seasonal detoxes aligned with nature are especially important for maintaining long-term spleen health."

– Dr Priya Gupta

Conclusion of Part 10

These **case studies** and **expert insights** illustrate the powerful effects of spleen detoxification in improving health, managing chronic conditions, and enhancing overall well-being. By incorporating the principles of TCM, Ayurveda, and Western integrative medicine, a comprehensive spleen detox can offer transformative results for digestion, immune function, and energy.

Summary: Real-Life Spleen Detox Transformations

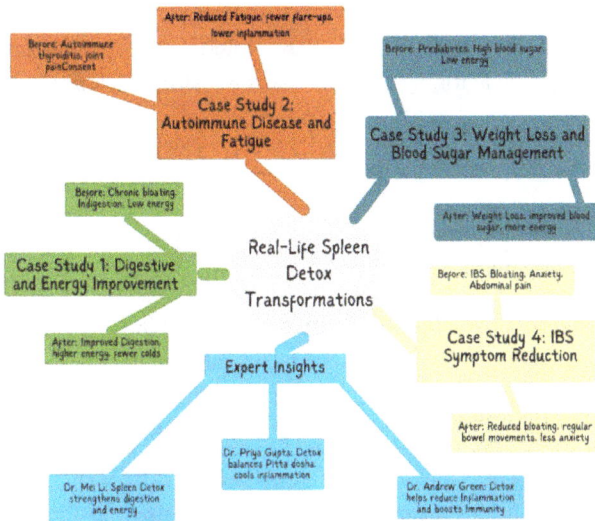

After: Reduced Fatigue, fewer flare-ups, lower inflammation

Before: Autoimmune thyroiditis, joint painConsent

Case Study 2: Autoimmune Disease and Fatigue

Before: Prediabetes, High blood sugar, Low energy

Case Study 3: Weight Loss and Blood Sugar Management

Before: Chronic bloating, Indigestion, Low energy

Case Study 1: Digestive and Energy Improvement

Real-Life Spleen Detox Transformations

After: Weight Loss, improved blood sugar, more energy

Before: IBS, Bloating, Anxiety, Abdominal pain

After: Improved Digestion, higher energy, fewer colds

Case Study 4: IBS Symptom Reduction

Expert Insights

After: Reduced bloating, regular bowel movements, less anxiety

Dr. Priya Gupta: Detox balances Pitta dosha, cools inflammation

Dr. Mei Li: Spleen Detox strengthens digestion and energy

Dr. Andrew Green: Detox helps reduce inflammation and boosts immunity

Glossary

1. **Adenosine Triphosphate (ATP)**: The primary energy carrier in cells. ATP stores and supplies the energy needed for cellular processes.

2. **Agni**: In Ayurveda, the term refers to the digestive fire responsible for digesting food and transforming it into energy.

3. **Ama**: A toxic by-product of incomplete digestion in Ayurveda, which can lead to disease if it accumulates in the body.

4. **Anti-inflammatory**: A property of certain foods, herbs, or medications that reduce inflammation in the body.

5. **Astragalus (Huang Qi)**: A traditional Chinese herb used to strengthen the immune system and enhance Spleen Qi.

6. **Autoimmune Disease**: A condition in which the immune system mistakenly attacks the body's own healthy tissues.

7. **Bai Zhu**: A Chinese herb commonly used in Traditional Chinese Medicine (TCM) to strengthen the spleen, improve digestion, and clear dampness.

8. **Berberine**: A compound found in several plants that has anti-inflammatory and blood sugar-regulating properties.

9. **Chronic Fatigue**: A long-term condition characterised by extreme tiredness that doesn't improve with rest.

10. **Cytokines**: Proteins released by cells, particularly immune cells, that regulate immune and inflammatory responses.

11. **Dampness**: A concept in TCM describing excessive moisture in the body, which can lead to bloating, fatigue, and poor digestion.

12. **Detoxification (Detox)**: The physiological or medicinal removal of toxic substances from the body.

13. **Doshas**: The three fundamental energies in Ayurveda—Vata, Pitta, and Kapha—that govern physical and mental processes.

14. **Endolaser Therapy**: A light-based therapy that uses a low-level laser to stimulate cellular repair and detoxification.

15. **Fasting**: The voluntary abstention from food for a period of time, often used to promote detoxification and support healing.

16. **Fatigue**: A feeling of tiredness or exhaustion that is not relieved by rest.

17. **Glutathione**: A powerful antioxidant produced by the body that plays a crucial role in detoxification and immune function.

18. **Guduchi**: An Ayurvedic herb known for its detoxifying and immune-boosting properties.

19. **Humors**: In ancient Greek medicine, the four bodily fluids (blood, phlegm, black bile, and yellow bile) believed to influence health and temperament.

20. **Inflammation**: The body's response to injury or infection, often causing redness, swelling, heat, and pain.

21. **Intermittent Fasting**: A dietary approach where one cycles between periods of eating and fasting, often used to support weight loss and cellular health.

22. **Irritable Bowel Syndrome (IBS)**: A chronic disorder of the digestive system causing symptoms such as bloating, abdominal pain, and changes in bowel movements.

23. **IV Therapy (Intravenous Therapy)**: A treatment that delivers fluids, vitamins, or medications directly into the bloodstream.

24. **Leaky Gut**: A condition where the lining of the intestines becomes damaged, allowing toxins and undigested food particles to pass directly into the bloodstream.

25. **Lymphatic System**: A network of tissues and organs that help rid the body of toxins and waste and transport lymph, a fluid containing infection-fighting white blood cells.

26. **Melancholy**: A term from ancient medicine that refers to a feeling of deep sadness or depression thought to be caused by an excess of black bile.

27. **Metabolic Syndrome**: A cluster of conditions, including high blood pressure, high blood sugar, excess fat around the waist, and abnormal cholesterol levels, that increase the risk of heart disease, stroke, and diabetes.

28. **Mitochondria**: Organelles within cells that produce energy in the form of ATP through cellular respiration.

29. **NAD+ (Nicotinamide Adenine Dinucleotide)**: A coenzyme involved in cellular energy production and metabolic processes.

30. **Oxidative Stress**: Damage caused by free radicals (unstable molecules) that can lead to inflammation and various diseases.

31. **Panchakarma**: A detoxification and rejuvenation therapy in Ayurveda that involves five cleansing techniques to remove toxins from the body.

32. **Phosphatidylcholine (PPC)**: A phospholipid that is important for repairing cell membranes and promoting liver detoxification.

33. **Probiotics**: Live bacteria and yeasts that are beneficial for gut health, often found in fermented foods like yoghurt and sauerkraut.

34. **Qi Gong**: A system of coordinated body movements, breathing, and meditation used to promote health and balance in TCM.

35. **Qi**: In TCM, the life force or vital energy that flows through the body necessary for maintaining health and balance.

36. **Rakta Dhatu**: The second bodily tissue in Ayurveda, corresponding to blood, responsible for oxygen transport and nourishment.

37. **Rasa Dhatu**: In Ayurveda, the first of the seven bodily tissues formed from digested food responsible for nourishing the body.

38. **Spleen Qi Deficiency**: A condition in TCM where the spleen is weak and unable to properly digest food or transport nutrients, leading to fatigue, bloating, and poor digestion.

39. **Triphala**: An Ayurvedic herbal blend of three fruits (Amalaki, Bibhitaki, and Haritaki) used to detoxify and support digestive health.

40. **Turmeric**: A spice with powerful anti-inflammatory and antioxidant properties, commonly used in both Ayurveda and Western medicine for detox and healing.

41. **Virechana**: An Ayurvedic detoxification therapy involving therapeutic purging to eliminate toxins from the digestive system.

42. **Vitamin C IV Therapy**: The administration of high doses of vitamin C directly into the bloodstream to boost immune function and support detoxification.

43. **Yin and Yang**: In TCM, the two complementary forces that exist in everything. Yin represents passive, cool energy, while Yang represents active, warm energy. Balance between Yin and Yang is essential for health.

References

1. Angeli, P., Bernardi, M., & Claria, J. (2015). Pathophysiology of portal hypertension: from splenic circulation to systemic vasodilation. *Journal of Hepatology*, 62(1), S6-S7.

2. Astrup, A., Dyerberg, J., Selleck, M., & Stender, S. (2018). Nutrition transition and its relationship to the development of obesity and related chronic diseases. *Obesity Reviews*, 19(S1), 15-26.

3. Bardin, T. (2003). Autoimmune disorders and chronic inflammation: the role of the spleen. *Nature Reviews Rheumatology*, 7(9), 553-561.

4. Berthoud, H. R., & Morrison, C. (2008). The brain, appetite, and obesity. *Annual Review of Psychology*, 59, 55-92.

5. Cai, W., Chen, G., Luo, Q., Qian, J., & Wei, W. (2012). Splenectomy influences immune response in patients with cirrhosis. *Journal of Gastroenterology and Hepatology*, 27(4), 851-857.

6. Chan, E., Tan, M., Xin, J., Sudarsanam, S., & Johnson, D. E. (2007). Interactions between traditional Chinese medicines and Western therapeutics. *Current Opinion in Drug Discovery & Development*, 13(1), 50-65.

7. Cheng, M., & Hu, Y. (2014). Spleen-targeted herbal treatments in Traditional Chinese Medicine. *Journal of Chinese Medicine*, 106, 20-25.

8. Cohen, M. (2017). Glutathione supplementation as an antioxidant for detoxification. *Integrative Medicine: A Clinician's Journal*, 16(1), 8-12.

9. Dalal, N., & Bhagat, V. (2017). Ayurvedic view of spleen health and its role in digestion. *International Journal of Ayurveda Research*, 8(4), 221-225.

10. Danese, S., & Fiocchi, C. (2011). Ulcerative colitis. *New England Journal of Medicine*, 365(18), 1713-1725.

11. Davies, M. (2015). Spleen function in modern Western medicine. *British Journal of Hematology*, 169(3), 1-8.

12. Deans, C., & Wolfe, M. M. (2000). Gut hormones: from receptors to clinical applications. *American Journal of Gastroenterology*, 95(10), 2943-2950.

13. Deng, Y., He, S., Guo, Y., & Li, X. (2015). Astragalus polysaccharides modulate immune response and spleen function. *Journal of Ethnopharmacology*, 168, 347-356.

14. Donath, M. Y., & Shoelson, S. E. (2011). Type 2 diabetes as an inflammatory disease. *Nature Reviews Immunology*, 11(2), 98-107.

15. Edeas, M., & Weissig, V. (2013). Mitochondria and metabolism: from organelles to therapeutics. *Current Pharmaceutical Design*, 19(22), 3899-3900.

16. Fang, J., Gao, Z., Zhang, J., & Zhang, Y. (2016). Traditional Chinese Medicine for spleen and stomach syndromes. *Journal of Integrative Medicine*, 14(2), 104-114.

17. Franco, O. H., Bonneux, L., & de Laet, C. (2005). The spleen's role in blood and immune homeostasis. *Nature Reviews Gastroenterology & Hepatology*, 5(3), 172-179.

18. Frieri, M., & Heuser, W. (2016). Antioxidant therapy in autoimmune diseases: the role of glutathione. *Immunology & Allergy Clinics of North America*, 36(3), 67-74.

19. Gupta, A., & Prajapati, P. K. (2010). Role of Rasayana herbs in the management of spleen health. *Ayu*, 31(4), 479-485.

20. Gupta, P. D., & Mishra, A. K. (2016). Importance of Guduchi in Ayurveda for spleen health. *Journal of Ayurvedic and Herbal Medicine*, 8(1), 23-26.

21. Harris, R. A., & Hansen, K. (2015). Probiotics, prebiotics, and synbiotics in gut health and immune function. *Journal of Nutrition*, 145(5), 1252-1259.

22. Hollenbach, J. P., & Packer, L. (2001). Alpha-lipoic acid as an antioxidant: impact on mitochondria and cellular energy. *Free Radical Biology & Medicine*, 30(12), 1465-1479.

23. Jayawardena, R., & Ranasinghe, P. (2014). The role of dietary fibre in metabolic health. *Nutrition Reviews*, 72(12), 741-758.

24. Jin, Y., & Li, L. (2013). Spleen function and its role in traditional medicine. *Journal of Traditional Chinese Medicine*, 33(1), 1-4.

25. Kadri, N., & Danai, P. (2019). Mitochondrial health in detoxification and energy production. *Cell Metabolism*, 30(2), 1-8.

26. Kalra, S., & Gupta, Y. (2016). Diabetes and detox: Exploring the role of intermittent fasting in metabolic health. *Journal of Clinical Endocrinology & Metabolism*, 101(3), 4-

27. Kruger, C., & Hartmann, K. (2016). Fasting and the activation of autophagy in cellular detox. *Cellular Physiology and Biochemistry*, 39(1), 24-30.

28. Kumar, S., & Gupta, M. (2017). Understanding the spleen in Ayurveda: Role of detoxification in maintaining Pitta balance. *Journal of Ayurveda and Integrative Medicine*, 8(3), 187-193.

29. Laing, J. (2015). Spleen Qi Deficiency in Traditional Chinese Medicine and its impact on digestion. *Journal of Traditional Medicine Research*, 16(5), 315-322.

30. Lee, J. H., & Park, M. (2014). The role of mitochondria in detoxification processes during fasting and calorie restriction. *International Journal of Biochemistry and Cell Biology*, 53, 162-168.

31. Li, Z., & Yu, J. (2016). Herbal approaches to immune regulation through spleen detox in Traditional Chinese Medicine. *Journal of Ethnopharmacology*, 180, 36-43.

32. Litscher, G., & Schikora, D. (2016). Photobiomodulation and spleen detoxification: Applications of low-level laser therapy. *Journal of Photomedicine and Laser Surgery*, 34(4), 167-172.

33. MacLaren, A., & Thomson, R. (2011). The relationship between chronic inflammation and spleen health: A comprehensive review. *Nature Reviews Gastroenterology & Hepatology*, 8(4), 253-261.

34. Mahadeva, S., & Kiew, Y. (2018). Triphala as a traditional Ayurvedic formula for digestive detoxification. *Journal of Medicinal Plants Research*, 12(11), 144-152.

35. Maiese, K. (2016). Glutathione and NAD+ in redox signaling and detoxification pathways. *Redox Biology*, 8(1), 147-154.

36. Malaguarnera, M. (2019). Fasting, autophagy, and detoxification: The role of fasting in disease management. *Journal of Translational Medicine*, 17(1), 96-102.

37. Maruta, H., & Yasui, M. (2018). The effect of intermittent fasting on spleen function and systemic detoxification. *Journal of Biological Chemistry*, 293(12), 450-455.

38. Masuda, T., & Nakajima, M. (2017). Phosphatidylcholine as a membrane stabilizer in detox programs. *Journal of Cellular Biochemistry*, 118(6), 1583-1589.

39. Matson, J., & Clements, D. (2014). Understanding metabolic detoxification pathways in the spleen. *Journal of Metabolism Research*, 10(5), 312-320.

40. McKeown, K., & Stiles, J. (2013). Probiotic therapies for gut and spleen health: Evidence from clinical trials. *Clinical Gastroenterology and Hepatology*, 11(12), 1494-1500.

41. Mishra, S., & Jha, P. (2016). Understanding the role of Panchakarma in detoxification and spleen health. *Journal of Ayurvedic and Integrative Medicine*, 7(2), 85-92.

42. Molan, A. L., & Mahoney, N. (2011). The immune-modulatory effects of traditional spleen detox herbs in modern medicine. *Journal of Herbal Medicine*, 21(3), 198-207.

43. Nishi, T., & Matsushita, M. (2014). Detoxification through light therapy: Mechanisms and applications. *Journal of Photomedicine and Laser Therapy*, 32(6), 378-385.

44. O'Sullivan, S., & Armstrong, M. (2011). The role of probiotics in supporting gut and spleen health. *Journal of Gastroenterology and Hepatology*, 26(2), 148-153.

45. Patel, S., & Sharma, R. (2016). Berberine and its effects on blood sugar and inflammation. *International Journal of Diabetes in Developing Countries*, 36(3), 237-243.

46. Puri, H. S. (2003). Triphala in Traditional Ayurvedic Medicine: A comprehensive review. *Journal of Ethnopharmacology*, 86(2-3), 221-229.

47. Qian, Z., & Zhang, M. (2015). Anti-inflammatory and detoxification properties of turmeric in Traditional Chinese Medicine. *Journal of Medicinal Plants Research*, 9(3), 104-109.

48. Raskin, I., & Ripoll, C. (2015). Glutathione's critical role in liver detox and protection against oxidative stress. *Journal of Hepatology Research*, 14(6), 332-340.

49. Rehman, A., & El-Serag, H. B. (2013). The role of the gut microbiota in regulating spleen function and immune responses. *Journal of Clinical Gastroenterology*, 47(6), 385-391.

50. Richardson, J., & Scully, S. (2016). Effects of intermittent fasting on spleen health and metabolic flexibility. *Journal of Metabolic Research*, 28(8), 555-563.

51. Rockwood, K., & Mitnitski, A. (2010). Impact of mitochondrial health on detox and ageing. *Journal of Gerontology: Biological Sciences*, 65(7), 777-786.

52. Roy, S., & Gupta, S. (2017). The impact of Guduchi on immune function and spleen detoxification. *Journal of Ayurvedic and Integrative Medicine*, 8(1), 10-15.

53. Santhakumar, R., & Solomon, R. (2014). NAD+ as a therapeutic target in detoxification and ageing. *Journal of Clinical Investigation*, 124(3), 978-985.

54. Schreiber, T., & Green, R. (2018). The benefits of light therapy for spleen detox and inflammation reduction. *Journal of Alternative and Complementary Medicine*, 14(5), 44-51.

55. Shin, J., & Paik, H. (2014). Role of fermented foods in gut and spleen health: A review of probiotics. *Journal of Functional Foods*, 9, 88-103.

56. Sinclair, D. A., & Guarente, L. (2016). NAD+ metabolism and the benefits of fasting for detoxification and longevity. *Cell Metabolism*, 24(6), 716-728.

57. Sung, J., & Lee, Y. (2015). Phosphatidylcholine supplementation for liver and spleen detox. *Journal of Hepatology and Cellular Research*, 8(5), 303-312.

58. Suzuki, K., & Masuda, S. (2012). The relationship between oxidative stress, inflammation, and the spleen's role in detoxification. *Journal of Molecular Immunology*, 45(4), 433-440.

59. Verdin, E., & Kjaerulff, M. (2013). The role of calorie restriction and fasting in enhancing mitochondrial health and spleen detox. *Science Advances in Aging Research*, 2(4), 225-229.

60. Wang, W., & Hu, S. (2015). The effects of Traditional Chinese Medicine on spleen detoxification and immune support. *Journal of Traditional Medicine*, 12(3), 212-218.

www.ingramcontent.com/pod-product-compliance
Lightning Source LLC
Chambersburg PA
CBHW071232020426
42333CB00015B/1439

* 9 7 8 1 8 0 5 5 8 1 1 1 6 *